MW01154706

Before Birth

A week-by-week guide to your baby's
development during pregnancy

Julie Currin MD

Copyright © 2015 by Julie Currin
All Rights Reserved.
ISBN: 1449570534
ISBN-13: 978-1449570538
Library of Congress Control Number: 2015918093
Celeste Publishers, Portland, OR

Illustrations by Thomas James

For Beth
and her blueberry

Contents

Introduction

Congratulations! As you read this book, and indeed as you go about your normal life throughout your pregnancy, your developing infant is accomplishing amazing things. While a mom's body changes quite a bit to accommodate the growing infant, the baby's body advances from two single cells into a completely separate, complex and fully functioning human being. All in 9 months—or is it 10 months?

The length of your pregnancy, as your obstetrician or midwife may have discussed with you, is officially 40 weeks, a full month longer than the 9 months we usually regard the length of pregnancy. This convention of the 40 week pregnancy is really to guide the obstetricians to more correctly predict when your baby is due. For most people, the timing of the actual conception is somewhat unknown, which would make timing the due date quite difficult and imprecise. So instead of relying on the conception date, doctors decided to time the pregnancy from an easier date to remember: the first day of Mom's last period. This is usually a date most women can remember, or count back on a calendar to figure out. Starting from that date, the doctor counts forward 40 weeks to determine the due date.

Now, obviously, you were not pregnant while you were having your period, even though that week officially counts as week 1 of your pregnancy. During week 2 of your pregnancy, the uterus is revving up again to prepare for a possible pregnancy. So pregnancy weeks 1 and 2 are fake weeks—when you are not pregnant, but doctors still count them as part of the 40 week pregnancy. Ovulation, or the release of an egg from an ovary, occurs at the end of week 2, which is the first step in a pregnancy. And so the beginning of the real pregnancy, the joining of egg and sperm, begins sometime in week 3. Therefore, the 40 week pregnancy is really about 37 ½ weeks of actual pregnant time, with an additional 2 ½ weeks of non-pregnant time added in by the doctor to more easily track the pregnancy.

Let's Get Started!

The 40 week pregnancy is the backbone of this book. Through this book, you will be able to trace your baby's development as it is happening, week-by-week. Believe it or not, not too long ago (like when I was in medical school in the early 2000's) OBs used a low-tech "pregnancy wheel" to calculate and keep track of a patient's due date and pregnancy progression. At each appointment, she (or he) would dial up the date of the last period and calculate due date and which week of pregnancy the woman was in. (This was often the job of the medical student shadowing that day.) These days, of course, everything is electronic, both in your life and in your doctor's. Most doctors are now using an electronic medical record, which automatically calculates and keeps track of the pregnancy weeks. And no doubt you have already calculated your due date on any number of Due Date Calculators available on the internet (if not, feel free to do a quick search now of "due date calculator" and you'll see a myriad of choices). Many of these sites will also offer to keep track of your pregnancy weeks and you can sign up for weekly emails. There are also apps that you can download to keep track of how many weeks pregnant you are, which can detail various symptoms of pregnancy, etc. And of course, you can simply mark the weeks off on a calendar on your wall or smart phone (or both).

Once you know where you are in your pregnancy, you can certainly flip to that chapter to get an idea of the appearance and new skills of your growing baby. The most dramatic changes happen in those early weeks, though, most likely before you picked up this book, so feel free to go back and review the trek your amazing tiny one has already taken.

Let's get started!

The Making of it All
Trimester One

The first trimester of your pregnancy is an amazing 11 weeks. In just under three months, a microscopic egg and sperm will become a rudimentary 2-inch miniature of the next love of your life—albeit without the bells, whistles, and working parts that will later enable her independence. This vital period is an incredibly active time developmentally, as a single ball of cells transforms into all of the major organs and the basic body form. Her brain, her heart, her face—even her fingers and toes—begin to take shape in this short period of time. Several of the important body parts will be in working order—her heart, for example, begins to beat in week five—while other parts take more time to develop. Through this unique window into your womb, we'll be able to see deliberate movement of her arms and legs, though she may not have perfected her wave quite yet. This is obviously a huge trimester, since everything that will make up the complex little person that you are so eager to meet gets started in these crucial months.

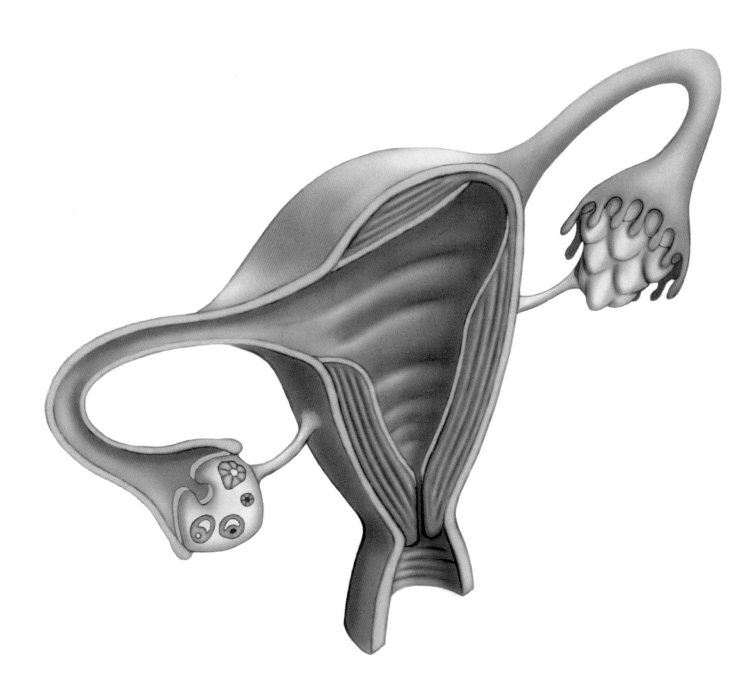

Before You Are Pregnant
Weeks 1-2

As we discussed in the introduction, weeks 1 and 2 of your pregnancy are fake weeks—days when you are not actually pregnant, but that count as a part of the 40 week pregnancy to make it easier on doctors to predict the due date. Since they came up with the convention, I guess they thought it fair to fudge a little here to make their lives easier. Even before there's a fertilized egg, your body is busy preparing for it, so let's pause for a brief overview of how your cycle works in any given month, and how your body has been preparing for these first 2 weeks of your "pregnancy."

During the course of a usual month—one in which you don't get pregnant—the first three weeks or so are spent preparing the uterus, or womb, in case you do get pregnant. For the first week and a half, this means thickening the walls of the womb; the second bit of time is spent secreting various hormones to make the womb most welcoming for a developing baby. The last week, if there was no baby made, it's time to clean house and start all over again—hence, your period. So, in this first week of your "pregnancy" this means taking a uterus with a thick, primed and ready wall from last month, scraping off all of that unused blood and tissue and ending with a thin uterus wall, in its resting state, as it were. As the uterus wall reaches its thinnest and most inactive state, we start into week 2, where your body begins to make more estrogen and the wall of the uterus first starts to thicken. This is called the Proliferative Phase, as the cells lining your uterus multiply, or proliferate.

The end of week 2 is marked by ovulation, which means that one of your ovaries releases an egg. This egg is able to survive for about 2 weeks on its own, but it is only fertile for a short period of time. If during that time, it does not run into any sperm, it self-destructs, the uterus gets the message that you are not pregnant, and we're back to cleaning out the womb to prepare for next month's cycle. If however, this little egg does run into a little sperm...well, then, it's time for week 3.

The Real Beginning
Week 3

Now that we are into the third week of your pregnancy, we can finally get to the part where you actually become pregnant—and for that we obviously need to bring together the egg and the sperm.

As the egg is released from the ovary, the finger-like fringe at the end of the fallopian tubes, or oviduct, bend and move, guiding the egg into the tube. Once inside this womb expressway, traffic slows. In fact, it takes an egg around 4 days to make the trip from one end of the tube to the other. Since the egg is only fertile for 10-15 hours after its release, this means that fertilization, i.e. the joining of egg and sperm, takes place inside the oviduct. And since sperm remain fertile only 48 hours, fertilization can only take place during the relatively narrow window of 48 hours before to 15 hours after ovulation. It's a wonder any of us are here at all, isn't it?

While the egg is floating in the oviduct, hundreds of millions of sperm are frantically swimming upstream in search of it. This is a very long and dangerous trip, with millions of casualties occurring in the several hour expedition. At the end of this arduous journey, the surviving hundreds of sperm find the egg at long last and attach themselves by their sticky heads. They still have several protective layers to dig through, but finally, one industrious sperm reaches the inner wall of the egg and dives right in. The outer covering of the sperm joins the outer covering of the egg and releases the sperm's genetic material into the egg. The sperm and egg are now one. The 23 chromosomes from the sperm mingle with the 23 chromosomes from the egg, giving this first cell its full allotment of 46 chromosomes, the same number of chromosomes found in each cell of our bodies. The fertilized egg at this point is much smaller than the period at the end of this sentence.

During the next 3-4 days, while the now-fertilized egg is still in the oviduct, the egg is not so much growing as dividing. Although it remains about the same size, the original two cells—sperm and egg—have now become 16-32 cells strong. These cells continue to divide as the egg reaches the uterus. It is while the egg is still floating around freely in the uterus that it begins

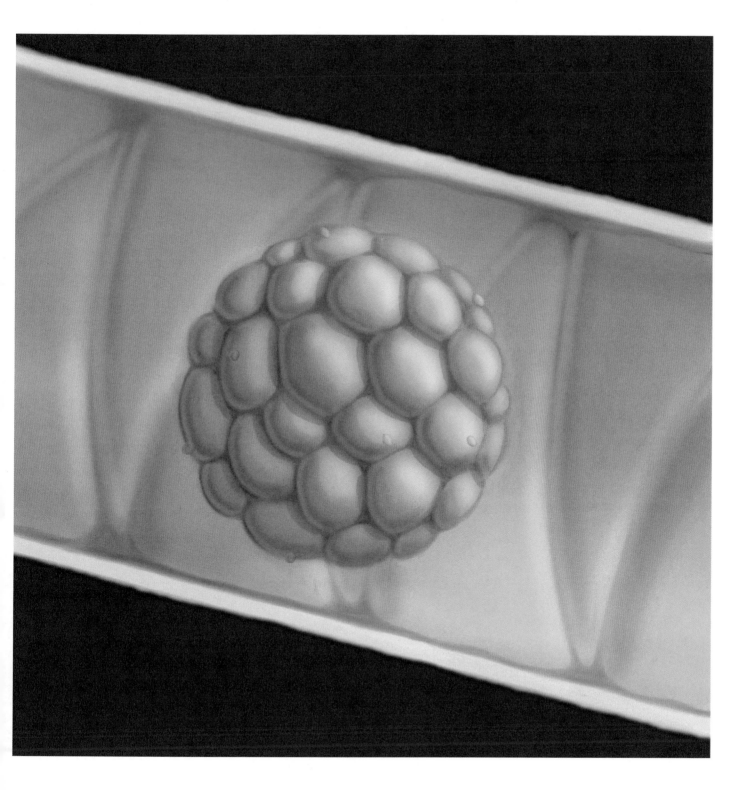

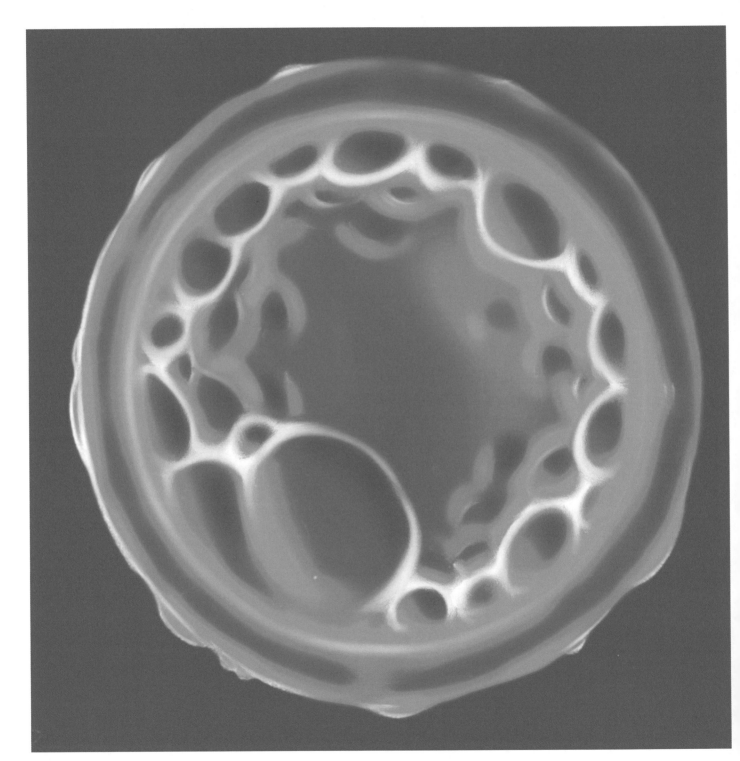

to take on any specific shape other than a ball—though it's still worlds away from looking like a baby. Fluid-filled spaces begin to appear between the cells of this tight little ball, and soon the cells separate into 2 separate layers with a fluid filled cavity between them—a thin outer layer and a clump of inner cells. Scientists, being scientists, decided to name your child at this point a BLAST-O-CYST, rather than Ball O' Cells (which is what blastocyst means). Now that she has this bizarre name and shape, she's ready to attach herself to the wall of your uterus. This is called implantation. The outer cells are quite sticky, especially the ones directly over the inner clump of cells. As this area begins to stick to the uterine wall, the cells of the wall and the outer cells of the blastocyst begin to merge together. We now have a fertilized egg, firmly attached to the uterus, from which it can get all the nutrients it needs—all in about 7 days.

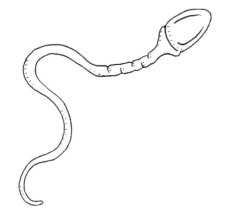

A slight variation in this process at one or two key steps can have surprising results. Twins, for example. Or triplets even. It is during this week that twins, triplets or more could have their start. This can come about in 2 different ways, at 2 different points in the process. The earliest of these variations occurs if the ovaries secrete more than one egg—this is how some fertility drugs work. Each egg can then become fertilized with a different sperm, forming entirely separate embryos and later babies. Since these babies came from different eggs and different sperm, they are not identical and in fact have as much in common genetically as simple siblings. If, however, only one egg is released and meets that one industrious sperm, twins can still be formed. During the initial dividing process, the fertilized egg can get a little overzealous and completely divide—into 2 entirely separate pieces, which each become separate blastocysts and develop into separate babies. These babies share all of their genes, since they came from the same sperm and egg, and are, therefore, identical twins.

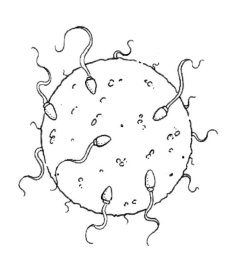

Two Layer Cake
Week 4

The fourth week is a busy time in blastocyst-land. The dominant activity at this time is splitting and layering, which sounds simple enough but is actually quite a complex process, difficult to explain and to understand; to complicate matters it is also a week full of big tongue-twisting words. As this process doesn't sound like very much fun on the surface, we're going to look at it from a more familiar angle—food.

At the beginning of this week, we have two main players—a clump of cells inside a mostly hollow ball, and a line of cells forming the edge of that ball. The first activity of the week is performed by the cells forming the outside layer of our blastocyst as they are busy worming their way into the wall of the uterus to firmly cement, or implant, the blastocyst into the wall of the womb. This completes the implantation process started last week.

The inner clump of cells is where most of the action takes place this week, though. Initially, the inner cells are all the same type of cells, collectively called the embryoblast. We're going to call it cake batter—in particular, this is a white cake batter (see recipe below). Half of this cake batter separates out (we'll pour it into cake pan #1) and becomes a separate layer, called the hypoblast. For the cake scenario, we're going to add some orange extract and food coloring, and make an orange layer. The remainder of the cake batter we'll make into a chocolate cake, which is called the epiblast. So now instead of having a mixture of similar cells, we now have 2 distinct layers, orange and chocolate. In the blastocyst, these two layers are still right on top of each other (think of our two layer cake stacked up with no frosting between them). Once the 2 layers have formed, they each begin to grow and swell (sort of, but not quite like in the baking process) and form into hollow balls, while remaining firmly attached to each other. The inside of the chocolate cake is called the amniotic cavity, and it will eventually make amniotic fluid which will cushion and support

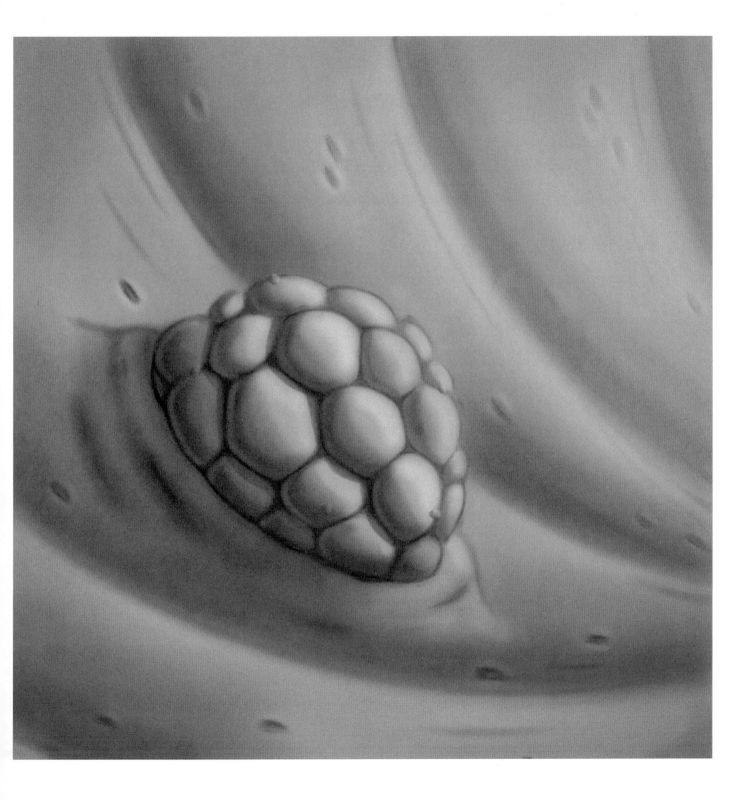

the growing fetus in weeks to come (and is what you'll see when your "water breaks."). The inside of the orange cake is part of what becomes the yolk sac, which forms the baby's first blood and blood vessels before disappearing altogether. Where the hollow chocolate layer and the hollow orange layer are touching, this is where your baby will develop.

Our cake, and our week, is not over yet. A third group of cells springs up from the epiblast, or our chocolate layer, and spreads out to completely cover our two-layer cake. This is like a chocolate frosting, which actually goes over the entire surface of our cake (though we won't make you frost the bottom of the cake) and is called the extra-embryonic mesoderm. This overzealous frosting then goes on to smear itself across the entire inside of the hollow ball of the cake, providing a second layer to the thick lining at the edge of the ball that holds our baby-cake.

At the end of this week, your baby is no longer a blastocyst, but has graduated to the name bilaminar disk—meaning two layer disk, or in our case, two layer cake. I suggest you celebrate with a piece of bilaminar disk cake and a large glass of milk.

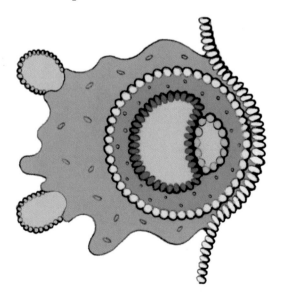

Bilaminar Disk Cake

3 cups flour

2 cups sugar

2 tsp baking soda

1/2 tsp salt

2 cups water

2/3 cups oil

2 tbsp white vinegar

2 tbsp vanilla

1/2 cup cocoa

1/2 cup water

1-2 tbsp orange zest

red and yellow food coloring (optional)

Preheat oven to 350 degrees. Coat 2 8x8 inch pans with non-stick cooking spray.

Combine flour, sugar, baking soda and salt in a large mixing bowl. Measure in water, oil, vinegar, and vanilla and mix until creamy (this is the **embryoblast**). In a small side bowl, combine cocoa and 1/2 cup water—mix well to avoid any cocoa lumps.

Remove 2 cups of the batter into a second bowl. In first bowl, add the orange zest to taste. Also add 2-4 drops of red coloring and 6-8 drops of yellow coloring until the batter becomes a pleasing orange color (**hypoblast**). To the second bowl, add the cocoa slurry and combine well (**epiblast**).

Pour the cake batters into the prepared pans.

Bake for 35-45 minutes, or until cakes are set. Allow cakes to fully cool before stacking and frosting.

Marmalade Filling (only included for flavor, does not exist in bilaminar disk)

2/3 cup marmalade

Heat the marmalade over medium heat until melted. Let cool 5 minutes before spreading.

Chocolate Buttercream Frosting (extra-embryonic mesoderm)

6 ounces cream cheese, softened

1/2 cup butter, softened

3/4 cup cocoa

2 pound bag confectioners' sugar

1/3 cup milk

1/2 tsp vanilla

Beat the cream cheese and butter on high speed until creamy. Add cocoa and vanilla. Alternate adding batches of milk and sugar, stirring until it reaches a spreadable consistency.

To assemble: place chocolate layer, flat side DOWN, on cake plate. Spread the marmalade over the top, almost reaching the edges. Place the orange layer, flat side UP, on top of the chocolate layer. Frost the edges first, using an off-set spatula, then frost the top. Enjoy with a large glass of milk!

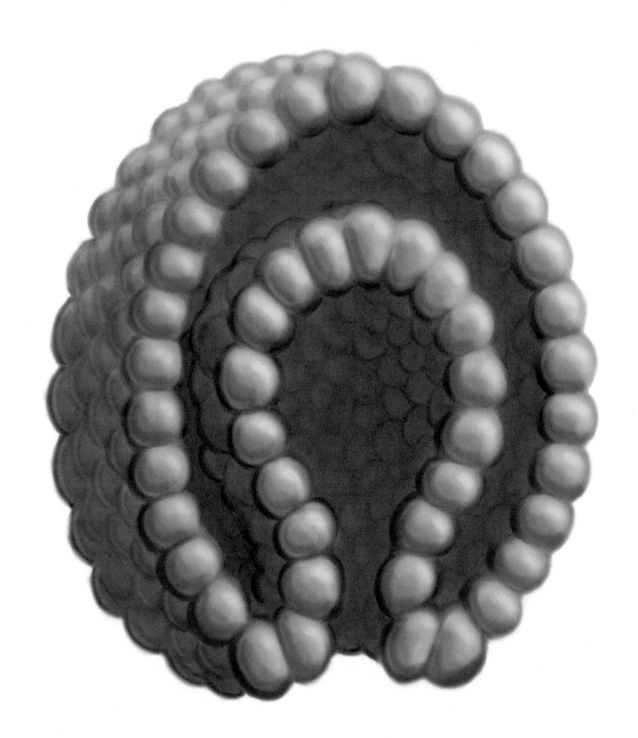

Three Layer Cake
Week 5

The main focus this week is the transformation from a 2-layered disk into a 3-layered disk—from a chocolate-orange cake to a chocolate-mocha-orange cake. This transformation occurs through a process called GASTRULATION, which isn't nearly as painful as it sounds.

The first step is the appearance of a tiny groove in the center of your future baby on day 1 of this week. Remember, your baby is forming where the chocolate layer and the orange layer touch. So, this groove appears on the inner surface of the chocolate layer just underneath where it joins the orange layer. As this groove develops and grows longer, a small pit develops at one end, surrounded by a mound of cells—sort of like an anthill with only one entrance at the very top of the hill. Strangely enough, this anthill has just determined which end of your little disk is going to become her head. Now that there is a new groove there, some of the cells in the chocolate cake layer begin to invade up towards the orange cake layer, forming a new layer. Since the cells originally came from the chocolate layer, we've made this cake layer mocha in our cake model. This mocha layer, as you can see from the recipe, is sandwiched in between the original chocolate and orange layers. The mocha layer is called mesoderm (literally middle layer), and its appearance forces a name change on the other 2 layers as well. Chocolate is now ectoderm (for outer layer); orange is now endoderm (inner layer).

During this seemingly easy process of gastrulation, your future ballerina has also grown so that at the end of this week she can reach a length of about 3 mm (about the size of a peppercorn) and is now referred to as a tri-laminar disk because of her 3 layers.

These new mocha cake cells, or mesoderm, are incredibly important in your baby's development. They migrate all over the place and become all sorts of important things—from bones and muscles to urinary tract and genitals. Speaking of genitals, during this 5th week, your baby starts working on those as well—and growing that all-important mouth. They don't look like much now, though. They are just two shallow depressions at each end of your baby disk. Of course, soon, like everything else, they will look completely different.

One of the most exciting developments this week starts around day 4 of this week. At this early stage, with your baby only a few millimeters long, we see the first appearance of what will be her brain and spinal cord. It starts as a small, flat plate near the head of the disk and expands backward toward the baby's backside, narrowing as it develops down the baby's spine. The broad section, the future brain, is already divided into 3 sections—fore-, mid-, and hind-brain. It will divide more later, of course, but the basic structure is already laid out. All of this has already started to develop, and you have just now missed that period you were expecting this week, so you might not even know baby disk is in there yet!

During this change into a three-layered disk, other important first steps are taking place. At some point this week, otic disks appear, which are the very beginnings of her ears. On about day 5 of this week, two parallel tubes begin to form in the area that will become the baby's heart, which is a horseshoe-shaped area above the forming brain (as the disk folds next week, this area will move into the correct spot well below her head). These tubes will join with the main blood vessel in the body, the aorta, which is also beginning to form this week. By the end of the week, this simple, primitive heart, begins to beat—keep in mind, your child prodigy is now about the length of the dash in this sentence.

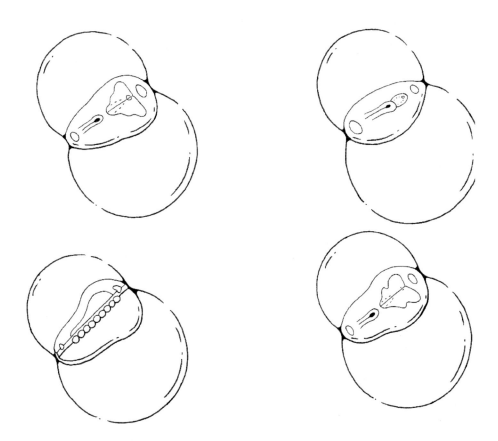

Trilaminar Disk Cake

Follow receipe for Bilaminar Disk Cake for the chocolate layer (**epiblast**), orange layer (**hypoblast**), marmalade filling, and chocolate buttercream frosting (**extra-embryonic mesoderm**). BEFORE ASSEMBLING:

Cut the chocolate layer horizontally in half. Mix 1 cup cooled coffee with 1 cup sweetened condensed milk. Mix well. Pour this coffee mixture over the cut side of the top half of the chocolate layer. Let sit 1 hour. (**mesoderm**)

To Assemble:

Place the chocolate layer (now the **ectoderm**) flat side DOWN. Place the mocha layer (**mesoderm**) on top, flat side DOWN. Press firmly. Coat the rounded side of the mocha layer with the marmalade. Place the orange layer (now the **endoderm**) on top, flat side UP. Press down firmly. Frost entire cake with the chocolate butter cream frosting (**extra-embryonic mesoderm**).

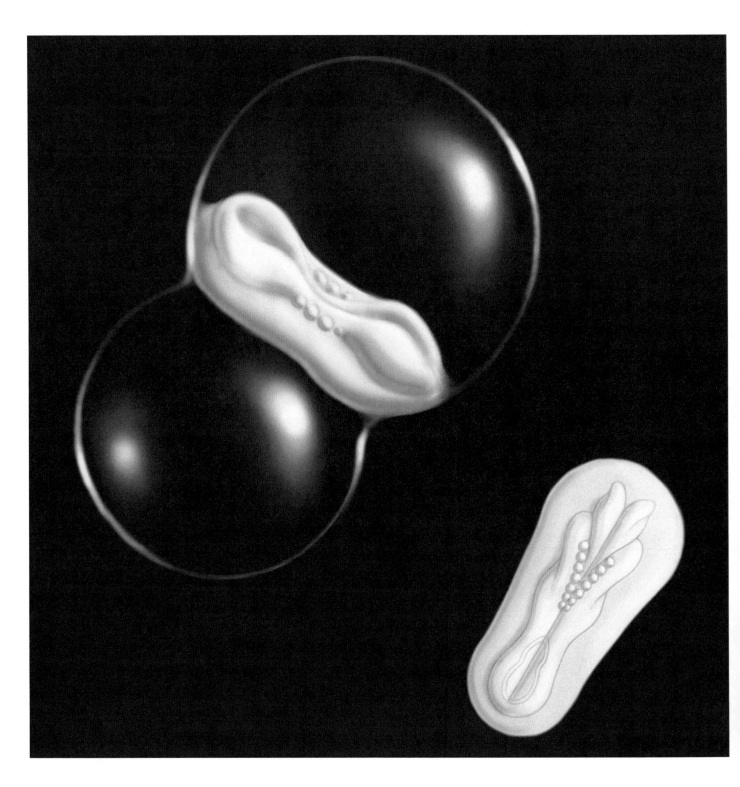

During week 6, we are witnesses to some dramatic changes in your future baby's appearance. Not only are we going to continue to grow in the all-important areas of brain and spinal cord, but we are also going to work on forming a primitive intestinal tract and becoming more three dimensional! Plus, we pass an exciting milestone, as this week your baby becomes a bonafide embryo. We also witness some astounding growth, doubling to tripling in size to 4-6mm, which makes him about the size of a cherry pit.

Last week, we walked through a process called GASTRULATION. This week it is time for NEURULATION, which involves the primitive brain and spinal cord plate that appeared last week. This plate that developed last week gets a tiny groove down its center. This groove serves as a hinge, so the plate on each side starts to fold in on itself and eventually forms a tube. By day 5 of this week, this is now a fully enclosed, hollow tube (we will fill it in later, as it develops into the spinal cord). We now have a three dimensional structure from which we can make a brain and a spinal cord. To go along with this newly-developing spinal cord, he is also starting to form the nerves that come out of the spinal cord to connect his brain to every part of his body, and the backbone that protects that vital spinal cord.

As this new tube is formed it starts to grow longer. Fast. This tube grows much faster, actually, then the rest of the disk. This is a very good thing, because this difference in growth-speeds forces your baby into the land of three dimensions. As the tube grows toward the head, it causes the top of the disk to fold over—the folded-over area will be where his face, neck, and chest will form. This explains why the heart that formed last week started out above the brain—after your baby-disk folds over, the heart comes to rest in the correct position. The tube also grows longer in the lower portion and by both sides, so that folding occurs along all edges. The folded over areas fuse

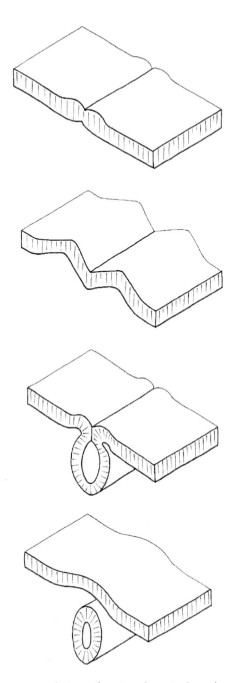

neurulation-- forming the spinal cord

together on the other side to form the front of your baby. This baby origami has just produced a 3-D figure, fully equipped with a front, back, top, and bottom!

As a result of all of this folding, the cells from the orange cake layer from last week, the mesoderm, have now become a tube. This tube connects the mouth depression, which now opens to form a slit-like mouth, with the urinary/genital area, and forms a continuous single tube from which the stomach, intestines, and other digestive organs will all start. As a matter of fact, almost immediately buds begin sprouting from this primitive tube that will become his stomach, liver, gallbladder, and pancreas. All of these organs are necessary for your little one to digest his food.

The lungs start from this digestive tube as well, though they have nothing really to do with digestion itself. In fact, the first lung buds appear in the very beginning of this week, splitting into 2 branches (one for each lung) by the end of the week. These guys will continue to branch through week 28 to form what doctors call the "respiratory tree" as its many branching passages resemble an upside down tree.

In a sense, the kidneys start forming this week as well, though what is really forming is a non-functional precursor to the kidneys. These fake kidneys are small, hollow balls that appear early in the week. They don't really do anything, and they disappear by the end of the week. They are important, however, since they are a required first step to making real kidneys. As these hollow balls regress, a second set of pre-kidneys show up to take their place. This week, these second kidneys are simply tubes and rods that will eventually connect with each other and with the outside world. This structure is not functional yet, but it will be in a couple of weeks, and is already working on splitting and branching off into smaller and smaller tubes.

The complex folding process this week also affects the brain and the heart. His brain folds and rotates, working itself from a straight tube into a convoluted structure bent in on itself in several places—more like an adult brain. Before the folding affects the heart, tiny divisions appear in the 2 tubes, beginning to form the 4 distinct chambers that make up the mature heart. The muscles of his heart appear on the first day of this week, which also marks the first day that blood begins to circulate through his body. By the next day, the heart starts folding into a fully 3-D shape, helping the two tubes merge into one and bringing what will be the four chambers into closer proximity.

Other important changes are taking place in your baby's appearance this week as well. During this week, 5 swellings emerge that will eventually join together to form the beloved face of your son or daughter, though honestly right now they just look like 5 lumps. The tongue also starts to form late in the week, as do the beginnings of the eyes and the internal ears. By the middle of the week, tiny buds begin to grow where his arms will be, and his legs begin sprouting by the end of the week. His skin is also changing this week, as it becomes 2 layers thick, with blood vessels forming in the deeper layer. His defining characteristic at this point in development, though, is a tiny tail, extending from his backside. As his arms and legs grow longer and look more like arms and legs, this tail will disappear, I promise.

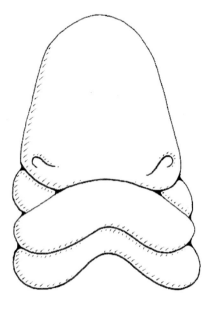

During week 7, our little embryo takes great strides towards looking more like her future baby-self. She continues to grow, so that by the end of the week she may be as long as 9 mm in length, measuring what is called crown-rump length—or the distance from the crown of her head to the roundness of her developing rump. At 9mm, she is about the size of a shelled peanut. One of her big accomplishments this week is spontaneous movement, though at this stage it is hardly more than twitching and much too slight to be felt by mom.

Her face is developing nicely from the 5 swellings that first appeared last week. The swellings around where her cheeks will be are growing down and in towards each other while flat plates over her nasal area appear and immediately start spreading out to meet the other swellings. In this nasal area, specialized nerves that will later enable her to smell begin to sprout and connect with each other. Filling in around the lower part of her face has provided her with a lower lip—long before you get to see it quivering as she cries out her demands. Her ears continue to develop and this week the external ears begin to appear. They start out as 3 swellings that appear on each side of her neck, which will grow together in the next few weeks. As her brain continues to grow and fold in on itself in the next few weeks they will make their way up to the sides of her head. Her eyes are also developing this week, with the appearance of the rudimentary lens as well as the beginnings of the nerve that will send visual signals to her brain—although these eyes first appear on the sides of her head, they, too will move into proper position—all propelled into proper position by her extraordinary brain growth.

On her chest, the primary bud of the mammary gland forms, which will be where her breast eventually develops. Both boy and girl embryos go through this step, as gender differentiation has not yet occurred, i.e. boy and girl embryos have so far developed identically. This is why men have

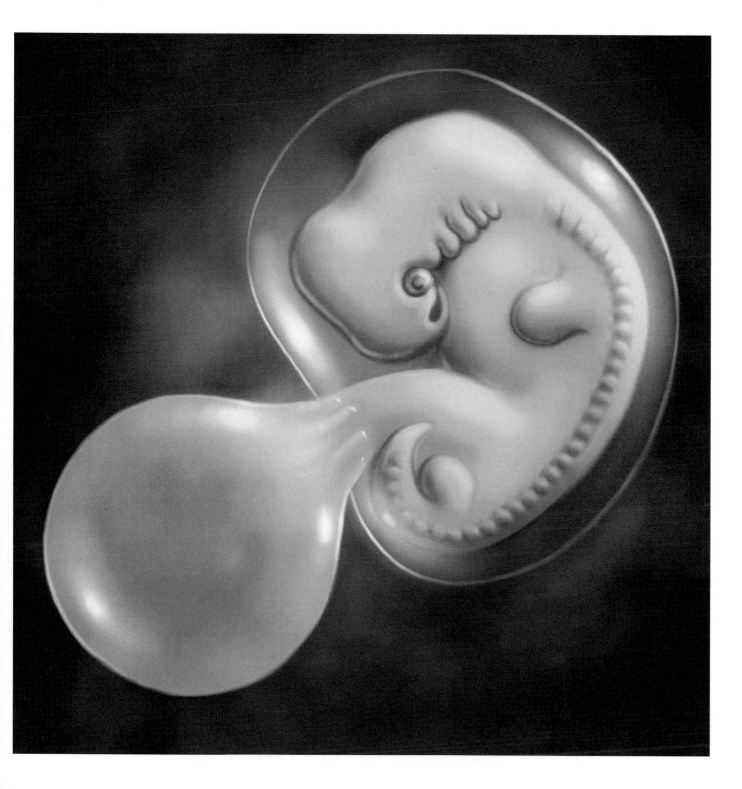

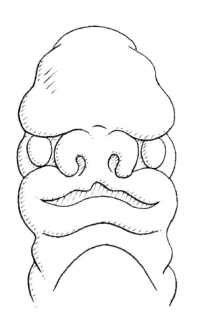

nipples, because at the point when nipples are formed, they've yet to start acting any differently then girls. Further down her body, her arms have developed enough that you can see where the hand, forearm, arm, and shoulder are going to be, and the bones begin to separate out as well. The legs trail behind a bit, but are now beginning to taper as they grow to where the foot will soon form.

Your baby embryo's brain has continued its complicated course of folding and flexing in on itself and has now formed a part of the brain called the pons, which is a part of the brainstem and is made up mostly of nerves connecting the rest of the brain to the nerves in the body. The right and left hemispheres first appear this week as well, starting out as bubble-like outpouchings from the front area of the brain. These are the main areas of the brain, the central post office where messages are received and sent out to the peripheral nerves throughout the body.

the infant's face and arm, still very early on in development

Not to be outdone, the heart has completed its transition from a set of parallel tubes to a four-chambered working machine. It still has much growing to do, but the form will remain essentially the same from this point on. The lungs have now fully separated into a right and a left lung, and have even begun separating into the distinct lobes of each lung, three on the right, and two on the left. There is still a long way to go before those will be operational. To protect all of these delicate organs, ribs begin to sprout from the backbone. They spread from the back, growing toward the chest, but won't reach their final destination for another 10 days.

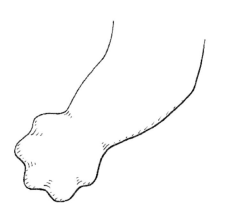

As we peek into her belly, we can see that the stomach is fast approaching its mature shape, as it grows faster on one side than the other, forming a pouch. Her spleen is now able to take over the job of manufacturing blood cells, and her small intestine is busy growing so fast that it begins to loop within the belly since there's not enough space to continue to grow straight. Lower in her belly, the very beginnings of either ovaries or testicles have been induced to develop, depending on the genetic cues sent out. This week, they are just two internal clumps of cells, called "genital ridges." These ridges sit near the bottom of her rib cage, but as they develop further they will head a bit further south. Though it is too early to tell the sex of the baby from the genitals, there is some activity going on down there. Whether it eventually develops into a boy or a girl, it starts out with a pair of swellings, called cloacal folds, on either side of a central membrane. A larger lump sits just above this membrane, called the genital tubercle (tubercle is a fancy word for lump). The diaper region has quite a bit of developing to do, but by week 14 it will be more than obvious (at least from our viewing point—it may not show up on ultrasound) what is waiting for you.

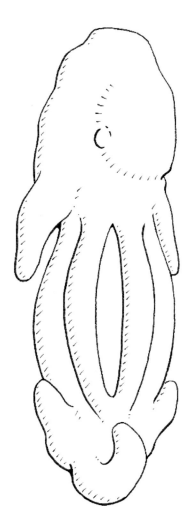

Blueberry
Week 8

While the basic appearance of your pride and joy remains at this stage a little hard to imagine, we are getting closer to a more baby-like look. He grows a bit bigger this week, perhaps reaching blueberry-size, up from his previous peanut, or about 12mm in length. This week, and size, holds a special place in my family—it was during this week in my nephew's development when he began to receive his nickname, now shortened to Blue. Be careful what you call your baby during the pregnancy, folks—old habits can be hard to break.

This week is marked in particular by many facial changes, all of which certainly help distinguish your fetus from a blueberry. His eyes progress further with the appearance of the color in the retina, which makes the eye now obvious on microscopic inspection. To protect these tiny, tiny eyes, folds start to appear in the skin around the eyes and form basic eyelids that spread across and cover the developing retina and lens. There will be no blinking yet, because these early eyelids fuse together to prevent any possible injury. They will separate after the eye is more developed.

The plates of tissue that formed last week in the nose area have now developed an oval pit in the center—it will soon separate into 2 breathing holes. Plus, the middle of the nose proper is being formed as two of the facial processes meet in the midline and join. The sense of smell continues to develop, with the appearance of the tip of the olfactory nerve, the nerve that carries smell sensations to the brain. As the mouth gets reduced from a wide slit to its final tiny width (which won't happen completely for a few weeks yet), U-shaped ridges arise on the upper and lower jaws. These are the very early preparations for the teeth that will erupt in a year or so. The external ear continues to develop, and now has gotten busy developing the canal that connects the external ear with the inner ear.

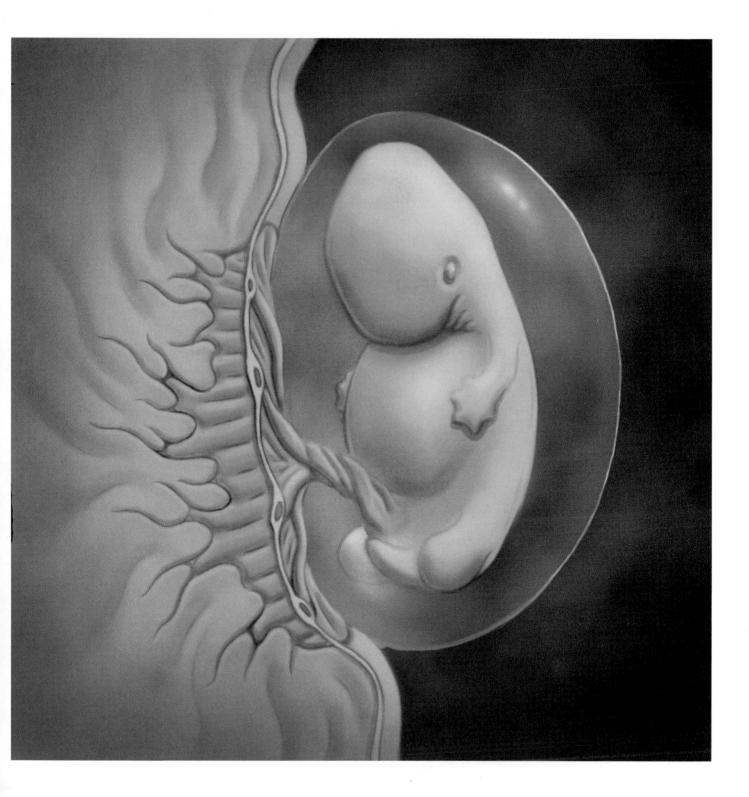

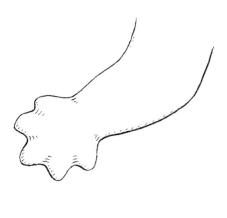

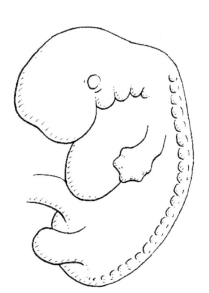

Our fetus is also making great strides this week in his arms and legs. This week, we can see the tiniest beginnings of his fingers and hands. Although his limbs may appear more like tube socks than anything else, if we look carefully we can see some flattening and widening at the hand-end early this week. The following day, four tiny rays or linear indentations appear, showing us where the fingers will separate out. While the legs lag behind the arms throughout development, by the end of this week, a flattened foot-plate is visible here as well. The bones are also starting to appear, though they first come in as cartilage, rather than real bone. By the end of this week, the cartilage versions of all of the arm bones, including those in the hand and wrist, will be laid out. Cartilage is a much softer, more flexible material, and so will begin to be replaced by firm bone as the baby continues to develop.

Lots of progress is also being made on the inside of our little guy. First of all, you may notice the prominent bulge in his chest—his heart is growing so much faster than the rest of his body that it sticks out conspicuously. In the belly, things are also getting crowded. The pancreas has now formed, from several separate pieces, and the intestines are getting long long long, and all the other organs in his belly are growing as well. It is getting so crowded in there, in fact, that the intestines push their way out through the belly button and into the umbilical cord in their quest for extra space. As they do this, they also start to twist around. At this point, your baby is still getting all of his nutrition from your blood via the umbilical cord, so the twisting intestines do not affect his nutrition-delivery system at all. And in a few short weeks, well before he needs his intestines for digestion, some space will open up, and the intestines will simply push their way back inside.

As he's working on developing his digestive system, he's also working on waste disposal—getting ready to fill your life with diaper changes. This week completes a process that has been going on for a couple of weeks in the hind portion of the digestive tube. It has been separating itself into the rectum (which you will get to know intimately in a few months) and something called the urogenital sinus (sinus just means cavity or open space). The urogenital sinus widens in one part, which will become the bladder, and narrows in the other end, where the urethra will form, which will take the urine from the bladder to the outside world (you will get to experience this little tube soon enough as well). The pre-kidneys that developed 2 weeks ago are now up and running, excreting small amounts of urine. While the mature kidneys' real job is to clean waste products from the blood, the placenta does this for the embryo. The kidneys' main job, therefore, while in the womb is to supplement the supply of amniotic fluid, making sure that your baby has enough fluid to float around in to keep it softly cushioned. While these pre-kidneys are doing the job for now, work is already in progress to form the final version of the kidneys, which will take over the urine job in a few weeks.

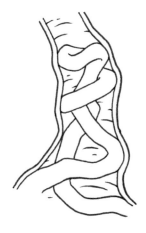

Finally, we return to the question of gender. The genital ridges formed last week have this week developed further clumps of cells, called primitive sex cords. This happens regardless of the ultimate gender of the baby. Next week, though, these primitive sex cords will have a starring role in making this baby a boy or a girl. Some related ducts appear this week as well, called Müllerian ducts. These ducts may have a very short life (if it's a boy in there) or may turn into her uterus or womb. For now, though, they are just itsy bitsy tubes, awaiting further instruction. We will catch up with them again in a few weeks.

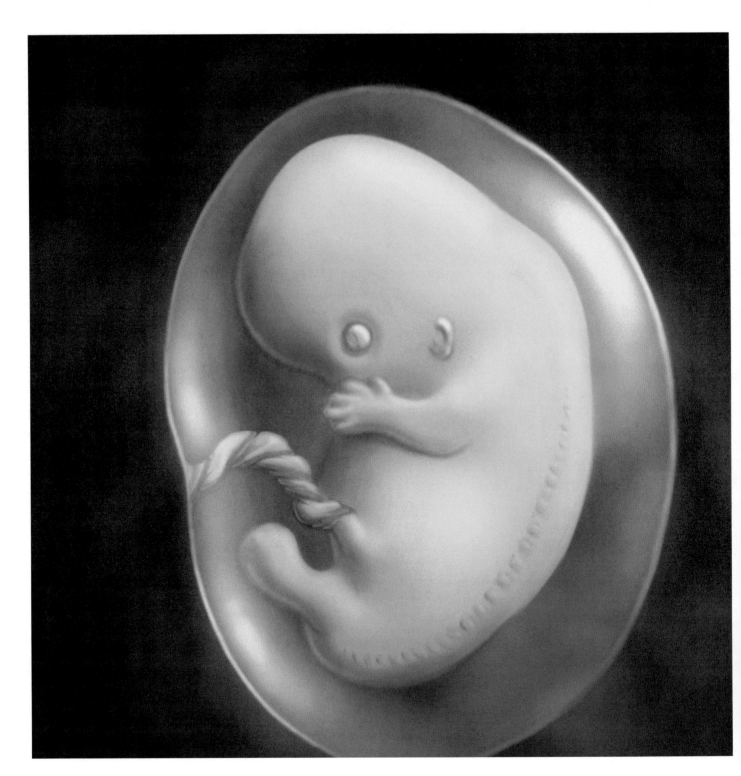

B o y   o r   G i r l
Week 9

During week 9, we are firming up the final face of this little one and witnessing some pretty good growth. By the end of this week, she will be up to around 20 millimeters, which is about the size of a blackberry. We also see big changes in her arms and legs. But the big excitement this week is that a boy starts developing differently than a girl. We will not be able to see what the gender is for some time, but the processes of differentiation start now.

Before we get to what boys start doing differently than girls, in both sexes we have to get rid of the membrane that has been covering the anus and the urethra. This membrane disintegrates, leaving 2 very important openings. The external appearance of boys and girls remains identical through this week, although there is still plenty of activity going on. The entire gender-forming process begins as he or she develops a pair of swellings called labioscrotal swellings (coming from the words labio and scrotal...any guesses on what these will become?). These swellings are the only change in the external appearance until week 15, when some big-time external changes take place. But on the inside, dramatic changes are occurring.

The process of becoming a boy or a girl starts with the baby's genes. A baby, as you probably remember, gets half of its genes from Mom and half from Dad. These genes are carried on 46 distinct chromosomes (23 from each parent). Two of these chromosomes are unique, and determine the sex of the individual. Mom is a woman because her two sex chromosomes are both called X (which is the letter they most resemble in shape). Dad has one X and one Y, which is what makes him a man. So, a girl gets an X from Mom and an X from Dad; a boy gets an X from Mom and a Y from Dad. This gene-donation process puts all the responsibility for gender squarely on Dad's shoulders. Therefore, in the legend of King Henry VIII when he beheaded several of his six wives because they were delivering girls only, he was being particularly unfair. (Perhaps he should have beheaded something a little closer to home!)

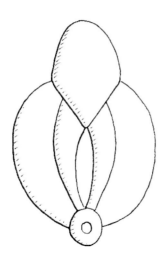

labioscrotal swellings (above) and early ear development as the three swellings come together to make one ear (below)

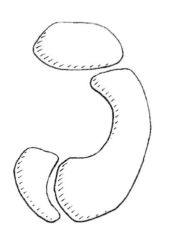

So this week, if you are having a little boy, this vital Y chromosome starts to cause a specialized protein to be produced called SRY (which stands for the sex-determining region on the Y chromosome). SRY is a very powerful protein. Its first move is to cause the sex cord cells, which are in the genital ridge, to become what are called Sertoli cells—these form into cords and, beginning at puberty, are responsible for sperm production. (We will talk more about Sertoli cells later, so remember that name.) At this time the sex cord cells round up and separate themselves from their surroundings to form testes. If your baby is a girl, and therefore has no Y chromosome, than the lack of SRY protein causes the sex cord cells to form ovaries instead of testes.

Also in this week, the facial development continues. Last week the lower lip filled in, and most of the nose pulled together; this week, as more of the facial swellings merge together, we can see the filtrum above the upper lip. The filtrum is the groove that you have between your top lip and your nose. Can you picture your tiny blackberry, already with this teeny tiny groove? So cute. Though teeth are a long way in coming (fortunately for those of you planning on breast-feeding), your child prodigy has already developed 10 little areas on each dental ridge where cells are proliferating. These cells are forming a total of 20 tooth buds, which will later pop up as her 20 baby teeth.

We also have some good progress on those ears. Although they are still hanging out on the sides of the neck, rather than the head, the three swellings on each side have become one perfect little ear—well, two perfect little ears, actually. The internal parts of the ear have been developing as well. The human ear is made up of three distinct areas: the external ear (for you to nibble), the middle ear (where kids get ear infections—this is the area behind the eardrum), and the inner ear (which helps with balance). Inside the middle ear, there are 3 small bones (incus, malleus, and stapes) which work together to relay sound. These are the bones that vibrate in response to the eardrum's movements and amplify the sound so it can be sent into the inner ear, where it is sent to the brain and detected as sound. These bones have begun to appear in our little one, though it is still too early for definitive hearing. The ears will continue to move up the neck and into proper position as the baby's face grows along with her brain.

Turning our attention to the rest of the body, the ribs that have been growing since week 7 have reached their final destination and have connected with the developing breastbone, or sternum. Her arms and legs are looking more and more like arms and legs, as grooves are now developing between the finger-forming rays from last week. Elbows are now obvious, and even the tiny finger bones are appearing in cartilage form. In fact, this week we can actually see real bone starting to form in the collarbone and in the upper part of the arm. In the leg, toe-forming rays are now visible and the bones are appearing as cartilage. She is also changing the position of both her arms and legs. Her arms begin to come in towards her body so that her hands lie across her chest. Her legs, which until now have been positioned so that the soles of her feet pointed up, begin to rotate and move in towards each other, bringing them into proper position with the soles of her feet ready to hit the ground running (hopefully not while she is still in there!).

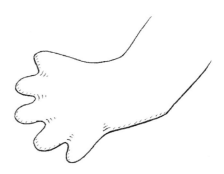

Wiggling Grape

With this week's advances in his face, arms and legs, the real humanness shines through your little one as never before. Plus, he grows another 10 millimeters or so, becoming a pretty good-sized grape. While he is still totally hairless, the beginnings of hair follicles appear at his eyebrows, along the edge of his eyelids, and on his upper lip and chin. His eyes are becoming more formed as the nerves that carry visual signals from his eyes to his brain are now solid and making connections where they need to connect. The muscles that allow his eyes to look right, left, up, and down are now formed, as well as the muscles he will need to open his eyes (though remember, his eyelids are still fused shut). His mouth has narrowed to reach its final width, and he now has cute little cheeks—almost ready for pinching (gently).

The big changes this week occur a little lower, though. As his arms and legs continue to develop, he is now able to wiggle his arms and legs (though this movement is still too slight to be felt by Mom). His fingers have developed little swellings on their tiny tips, which are called tactile pads, almost like those of treefrogs, only, of course, temporary in his case. His hands, which have mostly stayed at his sides, now meet each other across his chest and usually rest over his heart. His feet, similarly, are approaching the middle of his body as his legs continue to rotate inward. As his legs rotate, the bones in his legs begin to switch from cartilage to bone.

Just as his arms and legs are adjusting into position, so are the organs inside his belly. This week, his stomach rotates into the proper orientation with the outpouching on his left. And his intestines, though they are still bulging out into his umbilical cord, have now finished twisting around—they will be ready to move back into his belly in no time at all.

Remember those Sertoli cells? Our little boy made them last week from the sex cord cells. This

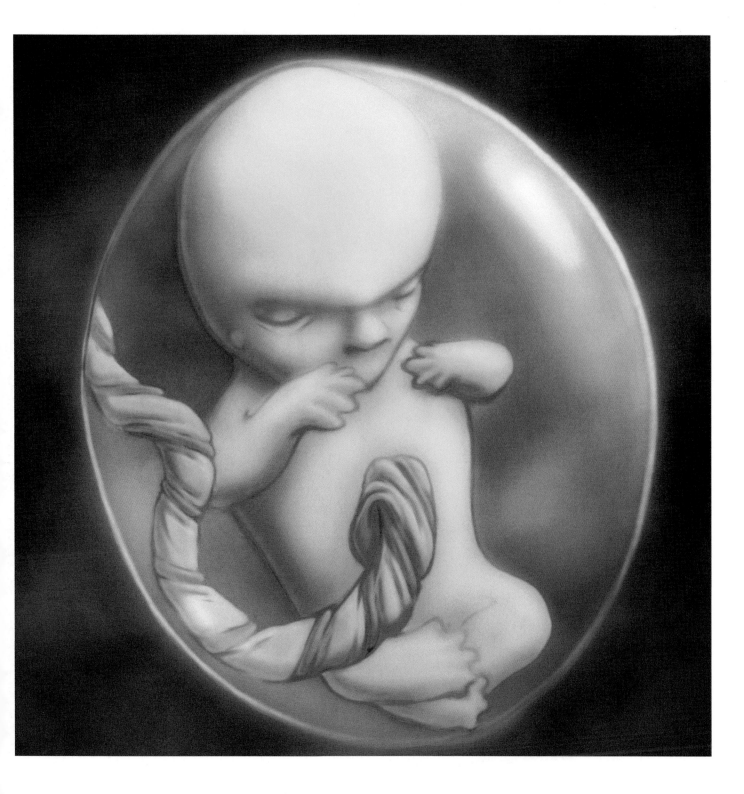

week, they are already busy making a hormone called anti-Müllerian hormone. As you may remember, Müllerian ducts first appeared in week 8, but they have not really done anything yet. As its name implies, anti-Müllerian hormone destroys the Müllerian ducts in little boys. If the fetus is a girl, and therefore does not have Sertoli cells to make anti-Müllerian hormone, the Müllerian ducts begin to join together to become the baby girl's uterus (or womb) and the oviduct (or fallopian tubes). Since we do not want little boys to have wombs, anti-Müllerian hormone takes care of removing the ducts.

Oh, and one last important change. By the end of this week, the "grape" loses its stem as Junior finally gets rid of that tail you've been worrying about. So put your mind at rest.

Big-Headed Cutie
Week 11

By the time you've made it to week 11, the final week of your first trimester, you have a pretty well-formed fetus, in that she looks much like a miniature version of the baby you will soon deliver. The biggest difference—other than the size—is that right now she has a very large head in proportion to the rest of her. Her brain has been developing very, very quickly, much faster than the body has been able to grow. In fact, right now her head makes up a full half of her entire body length. In the next trimester, the rate of body growth picks up, and she will lose this big-headed look. By the end of this week, she could be 40-50 millimeters, (about 2 inches) long, making her the size of a large strawberry. If you could peek inside (with a magnifying glass), you would see well-formed fingers and toes at the ends of her arms and legs and a tiny little baby face. She is still very skinny, though, since all of her efforts at this point have been aimed at developing new bits and pieces, and she has not had enough spare energy yet to beef up.

As the head is the focus of development and growth right now, it should not be surprising that the highlights of this week include the development of a new brain structure. The corpus callosum connects the right half of the brain to the left half. This vital structure begins to form this week, starting at the front of the brain and working its way toward the back.

Not to be outdone, her opposite end is developing new things as well. If we have a boy on our hands, the protein SRY which incited the Sertoli cells to form in week 9 induces another set of cells to form, the Leydig cells. Leydig cells are responsible for producing testosterone, which they can actually start to do in the next few weeks. Meanwhile, his testicles are moving into proper position. They start high up in the belly, so they have a long way to go. In fact, they won't reach the bottom of the belly/pelvic region for 3 more weeks. And then they still have one other big jump before they can rest in the scrotum.

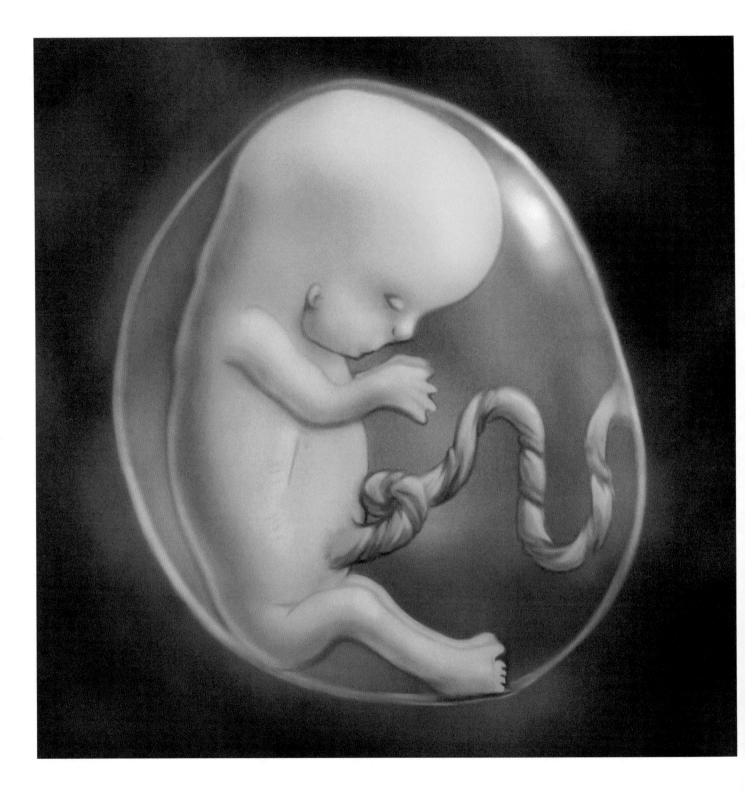

Testicles aren't the only migrating parts this week. In both boy and girl fetuses, the kidneys have been heading north, from low in the pelvis up to the low back. They are almost in their final position by the end of this week, though they are still not fully functional.

Growth and Fine-Tuning
Trimester Two

By the end of the first trimester, the form of much of our little one is already established. This does not mean that we have nothing left to accomplish during the second trimester. But the most obvious change will be in his overall size. By the end of week 23, he will have jumped from a mere a 2 inch golf ball to 7 ½ inches—about the length of a banana. He will also be putting on quite a bit of weight, ending up around 500 grams, or a little less than the weight of a can of soup. He weighs less than 50 grams at the beginning of the trimester, so he has quite a ways to go in the few short weeks. For the first time in his life, some of this weight will actually be fat, which helps round out his appearance. He picks up some color for his skin, and becomes able to keep warm (with the arrival of "brown fat") as well as cool down (as sweat glands form). He is also preparing for outside life in other ways, as he masters sucking and swallowing, and practices breathing movements. His arms and legs start to work, eventually even making themselves known to mom as his coordinated movements are finally felt. One of the most important milestones he will reach this trimester is gender differentiation, as boys and girls begin to look different during week 15. So even though the first trimester laid the foundation, there are still plenty of milestones left for him (or her!) to conquer in this one.

Crying and Peeing
Week 12

As expectant parents, you are likely looking forward to all the wonderful things that babies bring into our lives. Unfortunately, this week's developments highlight the less wonderful things that babies are famous for—dirty diapers and piercing cries. Neither of which do you need to worry about quite yet, but as these are such important life-skills, she starts practicing early. Also this week, we get a glimpse of the hallmark of the second trimester, which is extraordinary growth. By the end of this week, she could be as long as 61 millimeters, about the size of a kiwi fruit. This is the largest growth spurt to date, a staggering 20-50% increase.

If we look closely at her face this week, we can see some interesting advances. Strangely enough, even though her baby teeth are still a long way from erupting, much less falling out, this week witnesses the first appearance of her permanent teeth tooth buds. These tooth buds won't develop into actual teeth for several years, yet, here we are, just starting the second trimester and they are already starting to form. We can also see some interesting movement this week. By this time, she is able to open (and close) her mouth, and even stick out her itsy bitsy tongue. This is not meant as a rude gesture; rather, is a key part of practicing for the very complicated process that she must learn by birth—that of sucking and swallowing. Another vital process, breathing, is also being practiced, even at this early stage. We can start to see breathing movements by the end of the week. Even though she is nowhere near ready to take that first breath on her own, she is experimenting with the muscle groups required for this momentous event (which will almost immediately be followed by that marvelous first cry).

Also in preparation for exiting the womb, her intestines have re-entered the abdomen after spending the last 4 weeks or so sticking out into the umbilical cord in order to have enough space to twist around a full 180 degrees. The wall of the abdomen begins to close over the opening that allowed

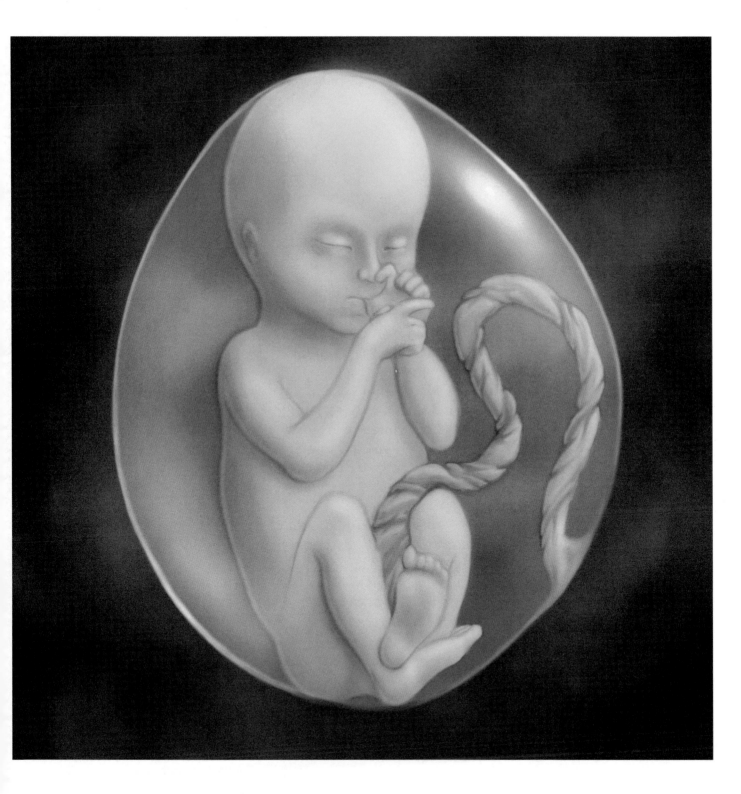

the intestines to push their way out into the umbilical cord, but this can be a very slow process and may not be completed until well after birth. This leaves many babies with a belly-button hernia, which is just the medical term for a small opening in the abdominal wall underneath the skin that can allow parts of the intestine to bulge out around the baby's belly button, especially while crying or pushing out her belly. As strange as it sounds, this area will continue to close up slowly and generally closes completely on its own in the first year of life, without any intervention whatsoever.

Lower in her abdomen, the final set of kidneys have now finally connected all of their tiny tubes together and become fully functional this week. They are taking over the job of producing urine that the temporary set of kidneys were doing up until this time. The temporary kidneys are regressing, as they are no longer needed. Take a moment or two this week to relish this time when your baby is peeing, but you don't need to change her diaper. It is, obviously, a short-lived luxury. Not too far from these kidneys, in boy babies only, the prostate gland begins to form. This gland buds off from the urethra and will eventually encircle it. In a few weeks, this gland will begin making hormones that lead boys down a distinct pathway toward making them look like boys, but for now it's just working on its basic structure.

One last new development of note: during this week, her fingers start to develop thickenings on the palm-side of each of her 10 tiny fingers. These are the very beginnings of fingernails, but don't worry—as soon as they start to form, they also start to migrate to the knuckle side of her fingers, where they are supposed to be. They grow pretty slowly, so we'll check up on their progress in a few weeks.

You might want to tell your fetus not to commit any crimes while he's in there—during these weeks he develops more distinguishing characteristics that could be described to a sketch artist. He also begins to develop miniscule ridges on his fingertips (and toe-tips) during week 14. Believe it or not, he is already forming his own unique fingerprints—so any criminal plans he may have had should now come to an end.

A tiny ring has been forming in his eyes for the last few weeks (this is one of those very slow processes). But, by the end of week 14, his iris is complete. Not only does the iris give your baby his eye color, but it also controls the size of the pupils to allow the right amount of light into the eye, expanding when it's dark and contracting when it's bright. Just as his eye color is coming in, his skin begins to change as well. He develops a new skin layer, sandwiched in between the pre-existing two layers, and begins to make melanocytes, the skin cells that produce melanin. Melanin is the hormone that gives your baby his color. Depending on the skin colors of Mom and Dad, he may have more or less of these color-producing cells—but however many he ends up with they are showing up now.

With all these new colors, he'd be easy to pick out of a line-up. However, not everything is coming through in color. His first hairs appear in week 14, but they are very fine hairs and totally lacking in color. They will cover most of his body, making him look a little furry. These hairs are mostly shed before birth and replaced with coarser hairs.

Also of note in these weeks, the cartilage in more and more of his bones has been turning into real bone. Now he has real bone in his shoulder blade and pelvis, for example, and even the tiny bones in his fingers. He will keep some areas of cartilage in each of his bones, as this allows for room to grow. The amount of cartilage gradually reduces throughout his childhood until he reaches his full adult height, when the only cartilage he has left will be in his joints, ears, and the tip of his nose (just like the rest of us).

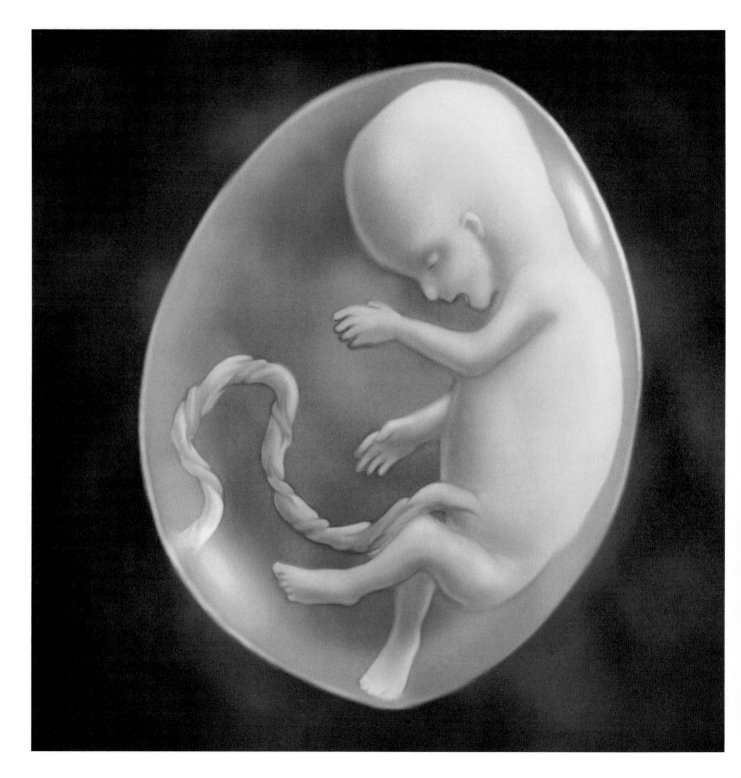

In little boys, the testes, which have been on the move trying to get as low in the body as possible, reach the lowest part of his body this week. They are still inside his pelvis, not in the scrotum just yet, but have reached what is called the deep inguinal ring. This is the ring, or opening, that leads into the tunnel that the testes will eventually travel into to find their final resting place in the scrotum.

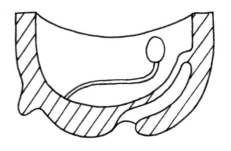

Little girls are also busy this week with their own girl-unique processes. She has been developing mammary glands behind the still-developing nipple from week 7. The mammary glands are multi-branching glands and will rapidly form several secondary buds off of the initial branches. At the same time, a canal has also been forming for the last few weeks called either the genital canal or the uterogenital canal. This canal will become her fallopian tubes, uterus, and vagina. Also during these last few weeks, her ovaries are being pulled into proper position. They were formed up near her rib cage, but by the end of the week they will be hanging out right where they should be in the far left and far right of her pelvis.

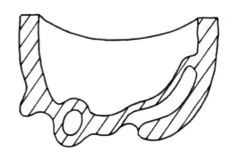

Even with all of these big external changes making your baby much more identifiable and unique in his appearance, growth is still not to be ignored. By the end of these two weeks, this precious baby can be about the size of an orange—and a pretty good-sized one at that. We are rapidly approaching that 100 millimeter mark (well, sort of, we're really only as far as 87 millimeters—or 3 ½ inches). He can weigh about 50 grams by now—about 1/6 of that weight is in his brain alone, which is still busy developing all sorts of complicated pathways and connections. As his body develops, he will begin to put on more weight as body fat and less as brain matter, so the percentage of weight that is his brain will decrease. This does not mean that he is losing brain power, but rather that his body is just trying to catch up. And his brain, of course, has lots of territory to cover, even after birth (but we'll save that for the next book).

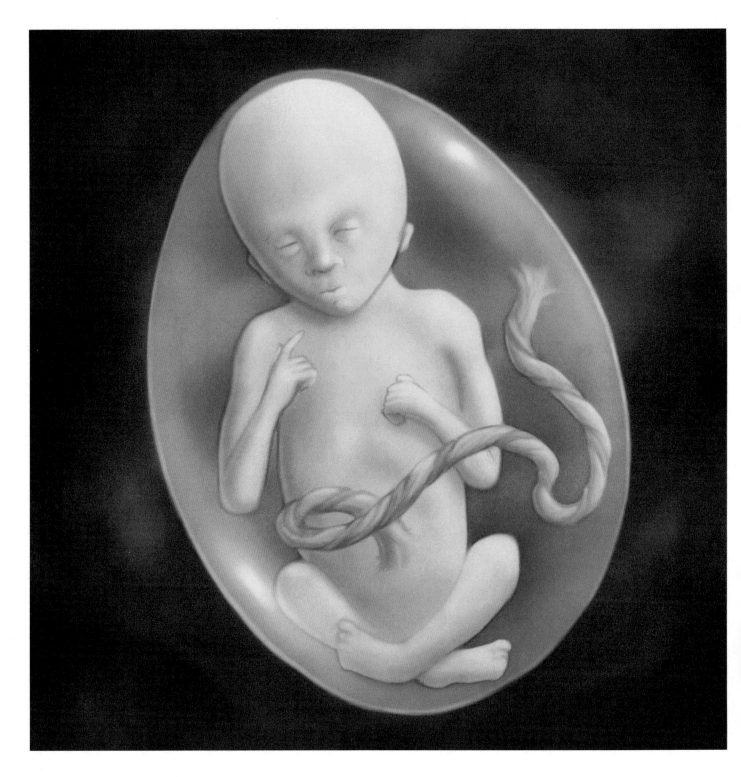

Jack or Jill
Week 15

This week stands alone as a special week. Only one significant event takes place this week, but it is one you have been waiting for. By the end of this week, if you had a magic window into your belly, you could tell if you should be painting that nursery blue or pink—if those are the sort of colors you're going for.

First, let's review things as they stand when we begin this week. In both genders, sex organs have been working on development, but have not differentiated in any visible way externally. Since week 7, we have been looking at a series of swellings and bumps. In the middle, there is a pair of ridges (called cloacal folds), which have a genital tubercle (or lump) connecting them at the top. On either side of these 2 ridges is a pair of labioscrotal swellings. All of these hills and valleys have been hanging out here for several weeks and are finally ready for a change.

In boys, the prostate gland budded off of the urethra two weeks ago. This week it starts secreting its hormone, which starts the whole external male cascade. The labioscrotal folds fold in together and join to form one larger swelling, which will become the scrotum. Remember that the testicles are still up in the pelvis, so right now this is just an empty sac. The cloacal folds also zip together in the middle, connecting fully with the genital tubercle up above. This tubercle, or lump, now combined with the two ridges, enlarges to form the penis, or what pediatricians sometimes call "his little weapon." (Remember to keep this covered as much as possible—you will be amazed at his pee-range.) We now have an obvious little boy.

Girls, of course, don't have a prostate gland to secrete any magic, boy-inducing hormones. So, nothing zips up into one piece. The separate folds remain, well, folds. The outside folds, the labio-scrotal swellings, become the labia majora, as the more central cloacal folds become renamed as

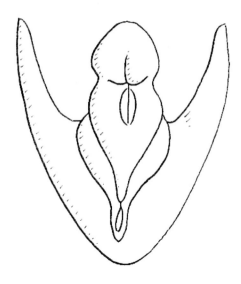

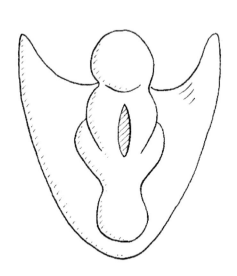

the labia minora. The genital tubercle in the center becomes the clitoris, completing her external reproductive system. We have ourselves a little girl.

Even though the gender of the baby is well-established externally by the end of week 15, you may or may not be able to know the gender of the baby by this time--or you may have found out a few weeks ago. Women who are at higher risk for certain genetic mutations, such as Down's Syndrome, may be offered a blood test early on in pregnancy which detects the baby's DNA floating around in mom's bloodstream which can then be looked at for a few specific genetic mutations. The sex chromosomes (XX vs XY) can also be detected this way, though if you want a surprise baby they can keep that part quiet. Amniocentesis is another method, used less and less now that the blood test is available. For amniocentesis, a doctor inserts a small needle into the uterus and removes some of the amniotic fluid around the baby to look at the baby's genes that are in the amniotic fluid. This is not done routinely, as it is not without risk, but it is the most definitive way to get information about the baby's chromosomes (and gender). Abdominal ultrasounds, or sonograms, are routinely done during a pregnancy and can at times reveal the gender of the baby with pretty good certainty. The penis or labia can often be seen by week 20, sometimes as early as week 16, but it depends to great degree on the position of the fetus at the time of the ultrasound. And there is still the possibility that you have a tricky little one in there who may be determined to be a surprise.

While our favorite fetus was developing all this new stuff last week, she was also busy growing. By the end of this week, in fact, she may be 120 millimeters from the crown of her head to her tiny little rump, which is about the size of a pear. She probably doesn't weigh as much as a pear, though, as she is just about 100-110 grams. This is about 3½ to 4 ounces, or roughly the weight of a quarter-pounder at McDonald's. Her brain accounts for about 15% of this total weight for now, although this proportion will increase dramatically in the coming weeks as her brain development really takes off.

This week we get to return to the development of her face, which has not seen much activity in the last few weeks. By the end of this week, she'll look much more human since her eyes have moved from their earlier position on the side of her head to their permanent position on the front of her face. In fact, if we could sit and watch her through our magic television camera into your belly, we could actually see her eyes moving around, like she is looking at her surroundings. Remember, though, that her eyelids are still joined together to protect her developing eyes, so she cannot really see much of anything, (not to mention how incredibly dark it must be in there) so she is really just practicing moving her eyes. She is also continuing to practice the vital and complicated process of sucking and swallowing. Though right now she is only swallowing amniotic fluid, which her kidneys will excrete as it moves through her system, in a few months this will be a life-saving skill.

We also see a significant change in her posture this week. Up until now, she has been curled up with her head bent over like she was staring at her chest. By the end of this week, however, she will be exercising those neck muscles, holding her head up and extending her neck. Of course, her neck muscles have a long way to go, and will not be able to hold up such a proportionally heavy head until well after birth.

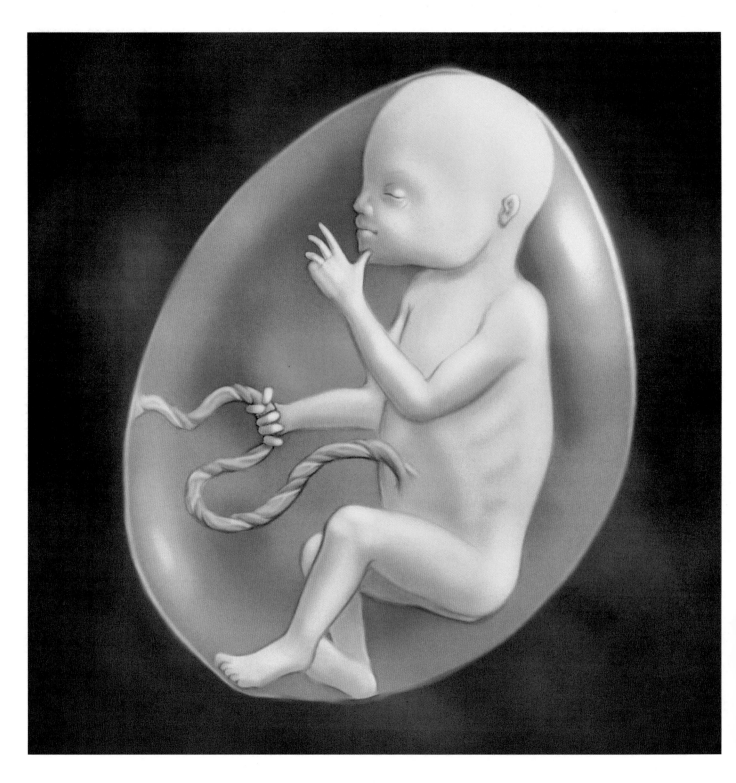

Not only is she checking out her place, but she is also interacting with it a little more. This week she can actually coordinate her arms and legs to move together in a purposeful way. What purposes she could have in there, I guess we will never really know. Now, don't worry that she is not bouncing around enough if you are not feeling any movement. It is really still too early for you to feel her punches and kicks. Keep in mind that her entire body is only pear-sized, so those feet and fists (and even that head) are pretty tiny. Speaking of tiny things, this week the tiniest of parts begin to form. The skin on her toe tips begins to thicken, which will form her toenails. Just like with the fingernails, which started to develop in week 12, these thickenings start out on the wrong side of the toes, on the very bottoms. As soon as they begin to form, though, they also start to roll around the side of the toes to land in their proper top-of-the-toe position.

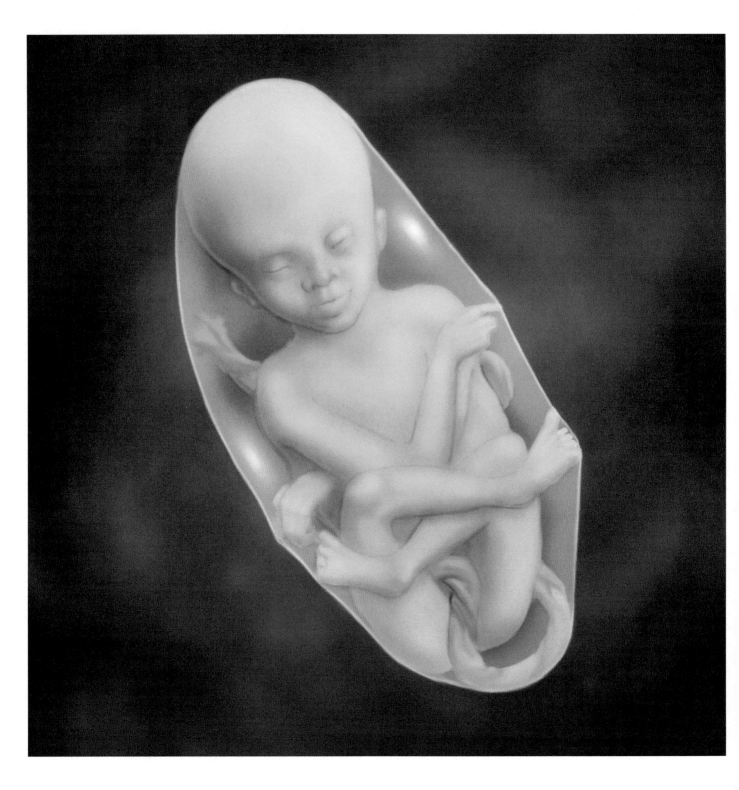

Doubles in Weight
Weeks 17-18

The seventeenth week is one predominantly of growth. You will notice that a lot more weeks are filled with "just" growth as we progress toward delivery. However, delivery is still a good ways away, and we do have more developing to do. And this "just" growth is a bit of a simplification. After all, in the last 4 weeks, your amazing child has doubled in length. When was the last time you doubled your length? Not to mention that he has nearly doubled his weight in the last 2 weeks. Hopefully, you have not had a weight gain like that since you were his size. With all of this growth, by the end of week 18, he will be around 140 millimeters (sweet potato-size) and 200 grams, which is almost half a pound.

Last week, we witnessed some significant face changes, particularly with his eyes. This week, it is his ears that change, as they plump out from the sides of his head, rather than lying flat against it. Between the ears, we have a good bit of brain development. In the last month or so, his brain has been incredibly busy forming complicated patterns of grooves and bulges, called sulci and gyri, respectively. By the end of this week, he should have a nice bumpy brain. His brain is growing very rapidly during this time and has actually started to bend into proper position. There are 2 large grooves that run horizontally from each of your eyebrows back towards your hairline, and as his brain makes this deep groove, it begins to grow and bend around it, forming what is called the temporal lobe of the brain, which lies just behind his (and your) temples. The temporal lobe is the area of your brain that registers sight, among other things. This is one of the first definitive lobes to form in the brain—several more will follow in the coming weeks as his brain continues to form these grooves and ridges.

In addition to growth, the eighteenth week is a time of branching and dividing. This branching occurs at two main structures that are still actively forming their multitude of tiny passages, the lungs and the kidneys. The respiratory "tree" in the lungs has been growing and branching into smaller and smaller air passages since the very early weeks when the right and left lungs first split. By this week, the airways have branched 14 more times and have now reached the smallest of formal passages, called terminal bronchioles. From here, they will develop airsacs, where the actual exchange of carbon dioxide for oxygen takes place. The kidneys have also been very busy dividing and branching. Each kidney now has between 14 and 16 lobes each. Even in this rudimentary form, they are functioning quite well, which helps keep a healthy amount of amniotic fluid for your little swimmer to float around in.

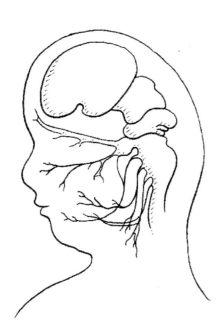

How About Some Heat in Here
Weeks 19-20

As we near the end of the second trimester, our little fetus has grown into a very lovely cantaloupe-sized fetus. Her length, remember, is only what is called her crown-rump length—that is, the distance from the crown of her head to the rounding of her rump. So the official sizing of 160 millimeters does not include the length of her legs, which of course would actually count in a real measurement of height. The reason for this omission is the position of the fetus inside. No matter how small she is, she still is not in a stretched out, reclining position, but rather she's curled up into a tight little ball, with her knees pulled up to her chest. This position, though probably quite comfy, is not ideal for measuring full-blown height, and so crown-rump length was introduced. (This is also the measurement they will take at all of your ultrasounds.) To go along with this increased length, she has also put on about 120 grams or so, bringing her up to 320 grams. This is a little bit more than a half-pound.

Though the fetus has been active in there for quite some time, moving her arms and legs even as early as week 10, she has been so small that the little bit of kicking and flailing has for the most part gone unnoticed, even by the most attentive and focused moms. This week, however, she just might work up enough energy to give you that first fully-felt kick in the belly you've been waiting for. Even if it does not happen this week, it will soon, so keep paying attention, and one of these days you will be startled out of your normal routine by a vague fluttering, the first hints of the activity that has been going on for quite some time now.

So far, our little girl has been focusing much of her attention on growing, and her little bit of weight gain is usually absorbed by her longer body. Because of this, she remains pretty skinny—fat cheeks and chubby legs come later. However, this week we do see the very beginnings of something called brown fat. Brown fat is actually quite important to the baby, because its job

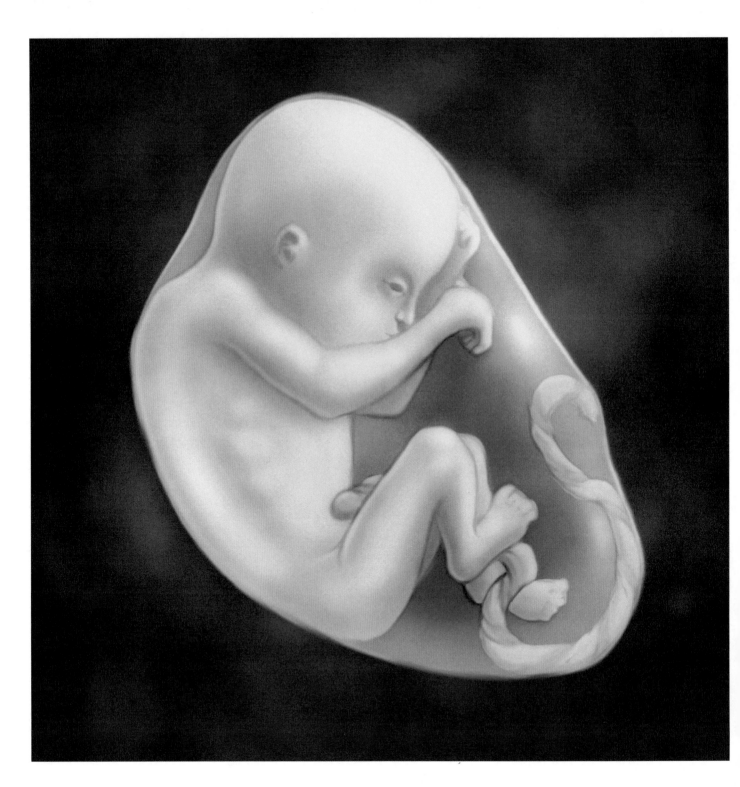

is to keep the baby warm. Brown fat actually is brown in color because of all the extra lipids it contains (lipids are just a specialized type of fat), and it has a lot more blood vessels and nerves running through it than the regular white fat. These extra connections allow a signal to be sent to the brown fat when the baby senses cold. After the cold signal is received, a special protein is released inside the brown fat that allows it to generate heat. When a baby is first born, brown fat may make up almost 5% of her body weight but will gradually decrease with age to disappear by adulthood. All this brown fat does not mean that you can take her out in the middle of the winter in just her diaper, but it will help her handle the cold underneath all those sweaters and blankets you'll bundle her in.

Let's Sweat, Baby
Weeks 21-23

In the last chapter, we saw a couple of seemingly unrelated changes. This week, the changes are mostly related to his skin. But first, let's take a sneak preview at his growth for these three weeks. By the end of week 23, he will be about 190 millimeters from his head to his rump. This is about 7 ½ inches, or the size of a head of cabbage. By this time, he could weigh up to 500 grams, which is just over one pound. One whole pound! It's taken us a long time to get here, but the weight gain from here on out is amazing, and he will be a normal newborn weight before you know it. Of these 500 grams, about 70 grams come from his brain alone, a whopping 14% of his entire weight. This percentage will decrease somewhat as he puts on some baby fat in the next trimester, but his brain will still be a major contributor to his overall size.

And now, on to his skin. With the beginnings of brown fat, the heat-producing fat, our little guy is starting to be able to generate some of his own heat. To balance this newest trick, sweat glands begin to appear during week 22. These glands show up over his entire body area, with only a few exceptions, which will ultimately allow him to cool himself off on those warm summer days. Also during week 22, his body becomes completely covered with soft downy hairs called lanugo. These hairs first started to form in week 14, and have now covered practically every skin surface. These colorless, fine hairs are usually shed by birth but may not completely disappear by the time of delivery. So don't be alarmed if your special baby has a slightly "furry" appearance when you first meet him; he just hasn't finished shedding his lanugo yet. Lanugo may linger for a few months but will be completely gone by the time he is 3-4 months old. Speaking of shedding, during week 22 that is exactly what is going on. The most external layer of skin is completely shed, leaving what used to be the middle layer as the new and improved outside layer. This is the skin you are so eager to touch. Just a few more weeks and you'll be stroking this softest of skins.

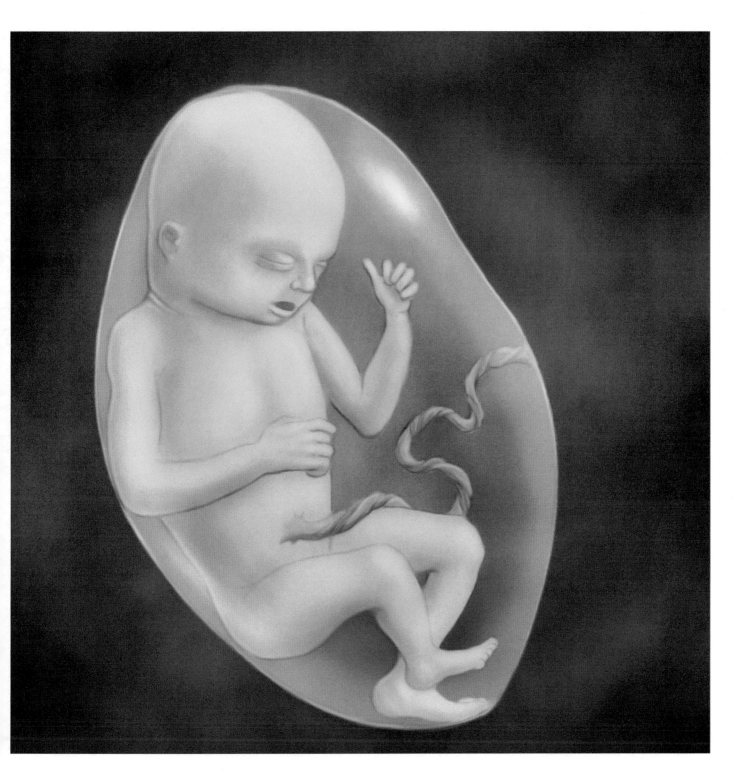

Last Minute Adjustments
Trimester Three

The last trimester is upon us, and we have quite a good bit yet to accomplish. All of these last-minute preparations help prepare him for life on the outside. Most importantly, his lungs need to get ready to blast their first shrill note…and to draw that nice quivery breath afterwards. His outward appearance changes quite a bit this trimester. His skin goes from red and wrinkled, to pink and oily, to the bluish pink of delivery. It also accumulates new glands (to be used in puberty, mostly) and all five million of his hair follicles. In boys, testes are on the move this trimester, while the fingernails and toenails of both genders are racing to reach their own finish lines before junior calls it a day and hops on out. One of the hallmarks of this trimester is growth—most notably weight gain (his, not yours, though they are obviously linked). At the end of the second trimester, he was a little more than 1 pound. By the end of this third trimester, he may well be over 7 pounds! This last spurt of weight helps round out what has been until now a skin-and-bones fetus. He's putting on his baby fat, and getting ready to leave that "fetus" label behind for good to become the beautiful baby you've been waiting so long to meet.

Wrinkles Already?
Weeks 24-25

As we begin this third and final trimester, our lovely little boy is weighing in at about 630 grams, which is almost 1½ pounds. Amazingly enough, he has gained an entire half pound in just the last two weeks, when it took him all of 23 weeks to gain that first pound. He is now about 210 millimeters long, a full inch over where he was last week and now up to butternut squash size.

His skin, which changed so much in the last few weeks, looks different once again this week. It is quite wrinkled at this point (though in a newborn, rather than a grandfatherly, kind of way), and is usually pink to red in color, and translucent. The wrinkles are mostly a preparatory move to accommodate the incredibly rapid weight gain he'll experience in the next few months before delivery. Most of the wrinkles disappear somewhat in the next few weeks as he puts on more weight and rounds out a bit (though he may still be a bit wrinkled at birth, which will allow for rapid weight gain in those early months). The color stays pretty much the same, though less red as he becomes less translucent with more advanced skin layering.

There is one more new trick that your tiny baby has learned this week—one that Mom may notice pretty quickly. Even though his eyelids are technically still mostly closed and joined together, he can have what is called a blink-startle response to noise. What this means is that with a sudden loud noise (or vibration) he can startle in the womb, which sometimes Mom can feel. He's not exactly blinking as yet, but he is having a blink response when he's startled, squeezing his eyes shut even if he cannot fully open them. It's a surprising world out there, as he's just beginning to discover.

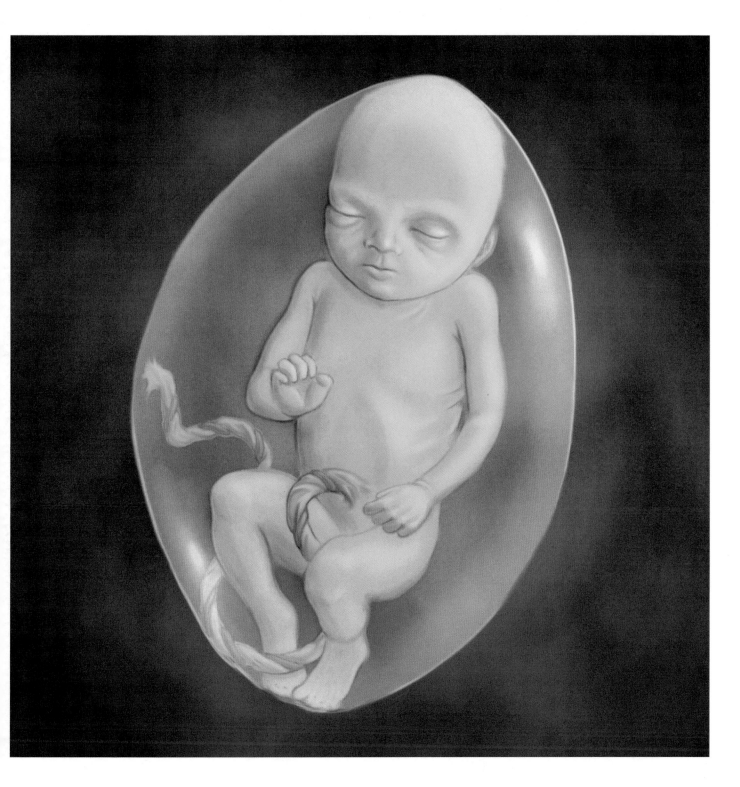

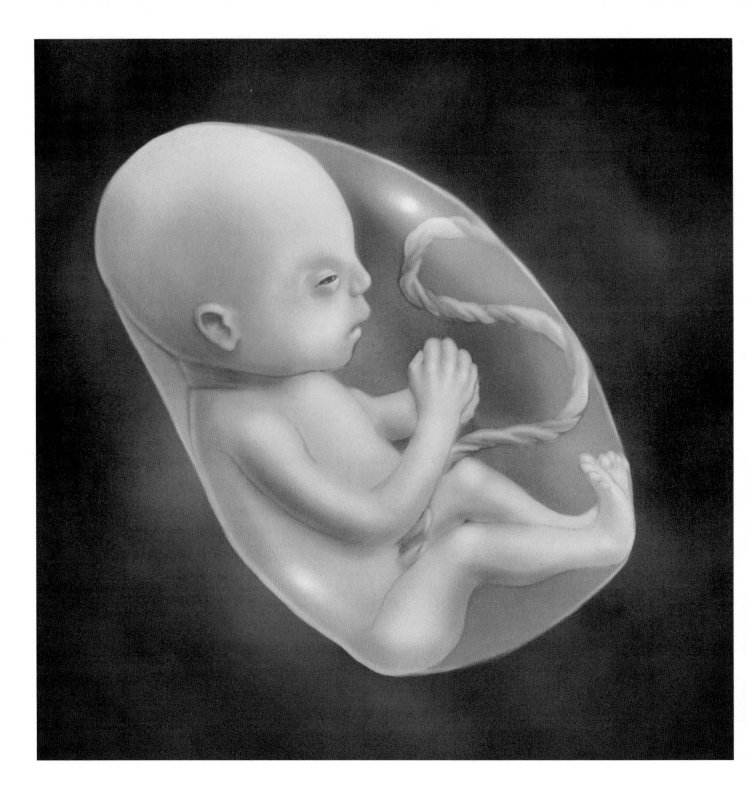

Waterproofing

We are continuing our steady march to the end of the ruler, and I am running out of food to compare her to! By the end of week 27, she will measure 230 millimeters, or 9 inches…or about the size of a medium carving pumpkin. She could weigh up to 1000 grams, which is over two pounds. She has really been putting on a lot of weight in the last few weeks. A good bit of it has been in her brain, which now could weigh 150 grams, 15% of her total body weight. (To put this in perspective, if an adult weighed 150 pounds, his/her brain would have to weigh 22½ pounds, rather than the 10 - 12 pounds it actually averages.)

Her brain has done more than just grow in size and weight these past few weeks. It has been busy making the basic divisions she will need as an adult. In particular, it has made two very large divisions, called sulci. The central sulcus divides the frontal lobe, which among other things contributes to personality, planning, and movement, from the parietal lobe, which is the center of feeling and sensation throughout the body. The occipital sulcus divides the parietal lobe from the temporal lobe, which has the areas for vision and memory. These are the main divisions of the brain, and leave her tiny brain looking pretty much like yours and mine.

The skin has been under construction for the last several weeks and is approaching its final form. One significant new development this week, though, is the appearance of sebaceous glands. These are the glands that secrete sebum, which causes acne in adolescents. Believe it or not, these glands are highly active in our little gal even now. The sebum they secrete helps create a waterproof, oily coating, which protects the new layer of skin that was only exposed a few weeks ago.

One last, but vital, development this week is the first secretion of surfactant from the lungs. Surfactant is an oily, liquid-like substance that coats the tiny branches and pouches in the lungs that help make the lungs easier to expand and deflate. In a way, it accomplishes the same thing as stretching a deflated balloon out before trying to blow it up. Without surfactant, lungs are stiff and very difficult to expand well enough to take necessary oxygen into the body. So while the lungs have been branching and dividing wildly for the past few months, generating miniscule branches needed for the exchange of carbon dioxide in the blood for oxygen, they are not functionally ready for the outside world until surfactant production is running efficiently. Even though the lungs start to secrete surfactant now, it will take a few more weeks until the complex process of breathing is really ready to be put to the test.

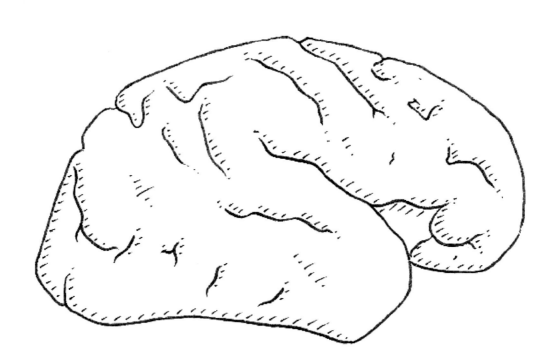

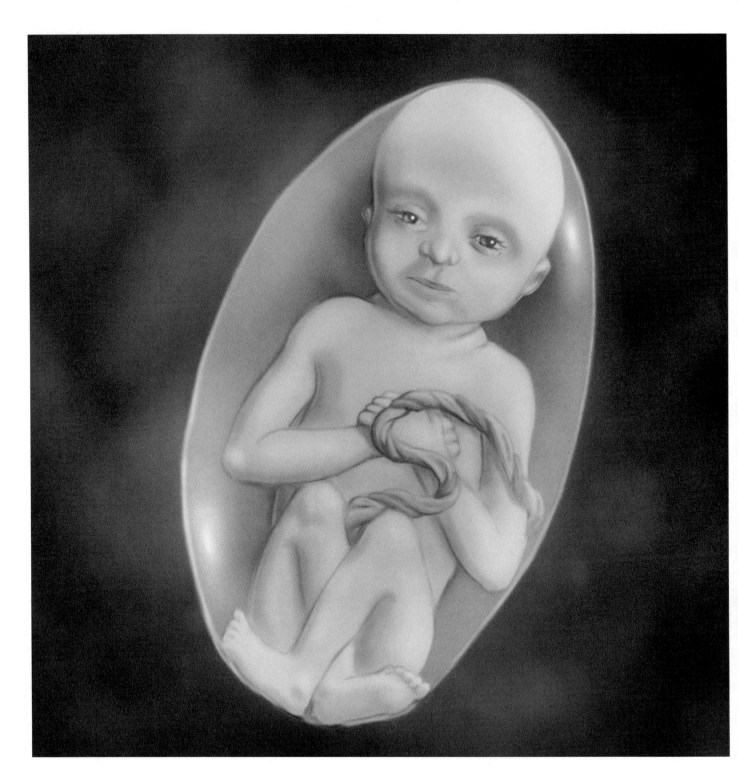

An Eye-Opening Experience
Weeks 28-30

We're getting ever closer to that golden due-date, which, by now, strangers on the street will probably ask you about—not to mention sales clerks and the produce guy at the market. Yes, you're getting big, and so is he. By the end of week 30, he could be 270 millimeters, which is 10½ inches, or about the size of a watermelon. He continues to gain good weight, coming in at about 1500 grams, which is a bit over 3 pounds. He is still keeping a mostly skinny figure, but will begin to fill out here shortly.

The painfully slow process of opening his eyelids reaches its end here. During week 28 his eyes are partially open, and eyelashes appear, helping protect the now vulnerable eye. In the next two weeks, though, his eyes are wide open and blinking. Strangely enough, as his eyes open, his ears close. His ear canals close up, self-implode, really. Almost as soon as they close, the outside opening of the canals begin to re-open, but the full length of the canals are not completely open until he's 9-10 years old. He may already have a good head of hair as well, colored similarly to Mom's and Dad's. His skin remains slightly wrinkled, but with the significant weight gain in the past few weeks is beginning to smooth out a bit.

His lungs continue to develop, beginning to be coated with the surfactant from the last weeks. They have now divided into the tiniest of branches, surrounding delicate tissue filled with tiny blood vessels. With this combination of small lung branches, tiny blood vessels, and surfactant to grease the surface, the lungs are now capable of breathing air. The brain has also developed enough so that it can direct rhythmic breathing, guiding the lungs and chest muscles into a proper steady rhythm. Hopefully, he won't need to try it out for a few more weeks, when everything has matured a bit—but he sure is getting ready to make his crying debut!

In these few weeks, the body is getting ready for departure. She's plumping up, protecting those delicate new organs with a nice fatty cushion. She now weighs as much as 2100 grams, which is more than a pound over where she was just a few weeks ago and just above 4 pounds. She is 300 millimeters long, which is practically a foot, though we are still not including her legs in her length measurement, which would be especially difficult in these later weeks as she gets even more scrunched up into the fetal position as she grows.

A lot of the activities going on for these few weeks are protective—preparation for her exit from the safety you have provided, into the harsh reality of life on the outside. In the last few weeks, she has made eyelashes and blink-startle responses to protect her eyes from debris. She is gaining fat to protect her organs and bones, as well as to keep warm. Her lungs are nicely developed now and she may be seen to be practicing breathing on ultrasounds as her brain is now well-developed enough to coordinate the many muscle groups necessary for this complex and vital exercise. During week 34, her tiny fingernails reach the tips of her fingers, as further protection. In boys, the testicles are working their way out of the abdomen, through a canal by his leg-joints, and into his scrotum. This, too, is a protective mechanism, as the scrotum will protect the testicles from the too-warm temperatures inside the body, which would prevent sperm production. Not that he needs to be worried about that yet, but this little guy is always thinking ahead.

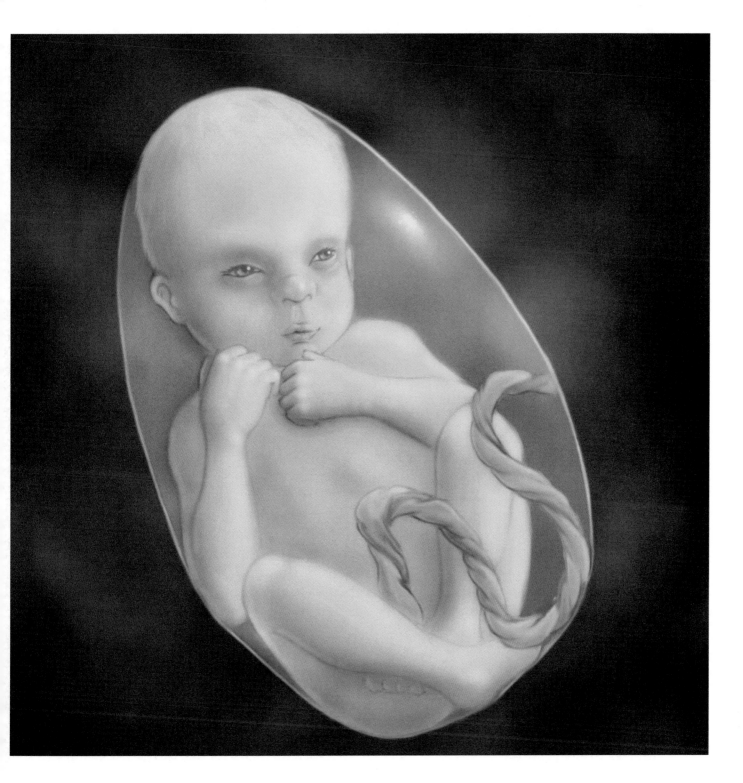

So, this is it—the final stretch. As you have been getting ready for him, he has been getting ready for you. By this point in his development, he is ready for life on the outside. These last 5 weeks (if he stays in for that whole time) are spent growing and growing and growing. Most of this growth is in his weight, rather than his length. While he may grow only another 2 inches or so, his weight may increase by as much as 3 - 4 pounds this month, an astounding 50 - 100% weight gain in just these last few weeks! This could leave us with a good 7 - 9 pound baby by the time of delivery. Over 10% of this total weight is in his brain alone, which is currently 25% of its future adult volume. Looks like we have one smart baby on our hands!

By week 36, our little guy is officially considered "full-term," if he were to decide to jump on out-a-there. This is because by this magic week, he is basically ready for life on the outside. The longer he stays in, the more weight he'll gain. For the most part, though, the rest of him is ready to go. His lungs will mature a bit more during this period, but they are ready to handle the difficult job of breathing by these last few weeks. By week 38, his skin is bluish to pink. At delivery he may look blue and pink, in particular a nice pink body with bluish hands and feet. He will get pinker after delivery, and may even appear red. This is partly because his skin at birth contains 20 times more blood vessels than it needs—the additional blood helps keep our little boy warm. As does the five million hair follicles he has, which is all he'll ever get. He begins to plump up after week 38, getting that round, baby look to his face and body. He is in decent control of that body of his now, too, and will spontaneously turn towards light and will firmly grasp anything placed in his tiny palm. Both boys and girls continue to have a prominent chest, and the area around the nipples may stick out slightly, almost like miniature breasts. This breast tissue is a response to Mom's hormones, rather than anything going on with their own, and will fade as your hormones gradually leave their bodies in the first few months of life. Boys should have both testicles fully descended into the scrotum by the time of delivery, as your doctor will no doubt check at his first few checkups.

So, here he is! Ready for the exciting life ahead of him. It's been a long road from those two tiny little cells, once such a small part of Mom and Dad. He took them and made them his own, turning them into the amazing creature you are just poised to meet: the little boy—or girl—who is about to steal your heart.

Your Newborn's Photo

Glossary

amniocentesis
A procedure in which a needle is inserted through the abdomen into the womb to sample the amniotic fluid that surrounds the fetus.

amniotic fluid
The fluid that surrounds the fetus in the womb.

anti- Müllerian hormone
A hormone secreted by the primitive testes in male infants that removes Mullerian ducts, thereby preventing the formation of female genital and reproductive structures.

aorta
A large blood vessel that carries blood away from the heart, down the trunk, supplying blood to the trunk and legs.

bilaminar disk
The term for the fetus at four weeks of development, so named because of its two flattened layers.

blastocyst
The term for the fetus at three weeks, as it is a hollow ball of cells.

cartilage
In developing embryos, the connecting tissue that is the precursor to bone.

corpus callosum
The structure in the brain that connects the right half with the left half of the brain.

chromosomes
The gene-carrying structure in a cell.

cloacal folds
The start of genital development; two ridges that will later develop into external genital organs.

crown-rump length
A measurement, commonly used in prenatal ultrasounds, from the crown of the head to the base of the buttocks. Used as an approximation of length since the legs are tucked up and difficult to measure.

deep inguinal ring
The internal entrance to the inguinal canal, which is the canal through which the testes travel to get from inside the pelvis to inside the scrotum.

ectoderm
The outer layer of cells on the trilaminar disk (the chocolate layer in our Trilaminar Disk Cake).

embryo
The technical term used to describe a developing infant from week six of development through week eight.

embryoblast
The cells that clump together in the blastocyst stage that will eventually form the infant.

endoderm
The inner layer of cells on the trilaminar disk (the orange layer in our Trilaminar Disk Cake).

epiblast
One of the two layers in the bilaminr disk (the chocolate layer in our Bilaminar Disk Cake). It later separates and forms the ectoderm and the mesoderm (or the chocolate and mocha cakes).

fallopian tube
Oviduct, or the tube that the released egg travels down that connects the ovary to the uterus.

fertilization
The joining of egg and sperm.

fetus
The technical term for a developing infant from eight weeks gestation to birth.

filtrum
The groove that extends from the middle of the upper lip to the base of the nose.

forebrain
The front section of the early developing brain.

frontal lobe
The front section of the formed brain; it deals with planning, reasoning, emotions, movement, and problem solving.

gastrulation
The process by which a bilaminar disk becomes a trilaminar disk.

genital tubercle
The precursor to the external reproductive organs, later turning into either a boy's penis or a girl's clitoris depending on the hormones released by boy or girl fetuses.

gyrus (gyri, plural)
The raised portions (or wrinkles) that make up the brain.

hernia
The bulging of intestines into an area that they do not normally bulge out into; can be through the belly button (very common) or into the scrotum in boys (less common)

hindbrain
The back section of the early developing brain.

hypoblast
The inner layer of the bilaminar disk (the orange layer in our Bilaminar Disk Cake).

implantation
The process of a fertilized egg attaching to the wall of the uterus.

labioscrotal swellings
The early development of the external genital organs, which will develop into either the scrotum or the labia.

labia majora
The outer folds of a girl's external genitals.

labia minora
The inner folds of a girl's external genitals.

lanugo
Soft, fine hair that covers a fetus towards the end of development.

lens
The part of the eye that focuses the images onto the retina.

Leydig cells
The cells in the testicle that produce testosterone.

mammary gland
The gland behind the nipples that produces milk.

melanin
The pigment that gives skin and hair its color.

mesoderm
The middle layer of the trilaminar disk (the mocha layer in the Trilaminar Disk Cake).

midbrain
The middle portion of the early developing brain.

Müllerian ducts
Ducts that form early on in development that later become a girl's uterus and fallopian tubes.

neurulation
Forming the primitive brain and spinal cord from a flat plate folding in and around itself.

occcipital lobe
The portion of the brain located at the back of the head that is responsible for visual processing.

otic disks
The primitive ear.

ovary
Female reproductive organ responsible for releasing an egg.

oviduct
Also called fallopian tube, this duct connects the ovary to the uterus and is what the released egg travels through to reach the uterus.

ovulation
The process of an ovary releasing an egg.

parietal lobe
The part of the brain located between the frontal and occipital lobes that is responsible for movement and recognition.

pons
The part of the brain located at the back of the head as part of the brainstem that is responsible for motor control and sensory analysis.

primitive sex cords
A group of cells that forms on the genital ridges and will later differentiate into either ovaries or testicles.

proliferative phase
The phase during a woman's menstrual cycle when the uterus is preparing for a pregnancy by thickening the uterine lining.

rectum
The end of the colon.

retina
The light-sensitive material at the back of the inside of the eye; it captures the light rays and converts them into electrical impulses that can then travel to the brain.

sebaceous glands
Microscopic glands in the skin that secrete an oily substance to lubricate the skin and hair.

sebum
The oily substance secreted by sebaceous glands that lubricates the skin and hair.

Sertoli cells
The cells in the testicle that are responsible for sperm production.

SRY
Named for the sex-determining region on the Y chromosome, this protein stimulates the primitive sex cord cells to form into Sertoli cells, which starts a cascade that causes boy fetuses to develop male reproductive organs.

sulcus (sulci, plural)
The grooves between the gyri in the brain.

surfactant
A slimy substance that covers the lungs late in the pregnancy to reduce the surface tension, allowing the lungs to expand easily when the baby breathes.

temporal lobe
The part of the brain located behind the temples, responsible for memory and language functions.

terminal bronchioles
The smallest and last branching of the respiratory tubing system.

trilaminar disk
A five week embryo, made up of three layers, the ectoderm, mesoderm, and endoderm.

urethra
The tube that connects the bladder to the outside world, allowing it to empty.

uterogenital canal
The precursor to a girl's vagina, uterus, and fallopian tubes.

urogenital sinus
The precursor to the bladder and urethra.

uterus
The womb

yolk sac
A sac that is attached to an embryo early in development that provides the embryo with needed blood and nutrition until it develops its own circulatory system.

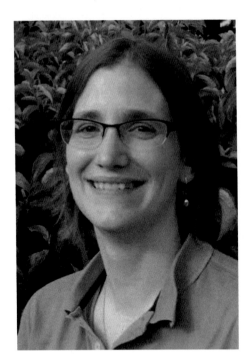

Dr. Julie Currin grew up in West Virginia, the youngest of 4 children, in a house full of books and storytelling, where she developed a love of language and learning at a young age. She graduated from Washington University in St. Louis with a degree in English while on the pre-med track and then returned to her home state to start her medical school training. After 2 years, Currin transferred to Brown University School of Medicine so that she could marry her college sweetheart who was attending graduate school in Rhode Island. It was during this time, while her oldest sister was pregnant with her first child, that she became aware of the gap in available books for expectant moms. Most pregnancy books focused on the changes in the mother's body, with only a sentence or 2 about the changes going on with the developing baby. Taking her knowledge of embryology and translating it into a fun and accessible forum for her sister turned into a fully illustrated book, which then sat completed on the back burner while Currin's professional and personal life blossomed. It wasn't until taking maternity leave for her third son that the book once again rose to the forefront and became widely available. Dr. Currin is currently a busy mom to 3 delightful boys and a practicing pediatrician in Portland, Oregon.

Made in the USA
Monee, IL
28 December 2020

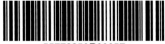
55772850R00057